# Trends in Men's Health

*Editor*

BRENT MACWILLIAMS

# NURSING CLINICS
# OF NORTH AMERICA

www.nursing.theclinics.com

*Consulting Editor*
BENJAMIN SMALLHEER

December 2023 • Volume 58 • Number 4

**ELSEVIER**

1600 John F. Kennedy Boulevard • Suite 1800 • Philadelphia, Pennsylvania, 19103-2899

http://www.theclinics.com

**NURSING CLINICS OF NORTH AMERICA Volume 58, Number 4**
**December 2023 ISSN 0029-6465, ISBN-13: 978-0-323-94031-3**

Editor: Kerry Holland
Developmental Editor: Isha Singh

*Nursing Clinics of North America* (ISSN 0029-6465) is published quarterly by Elsevier Inc., 360 Park Avenue South, New York, NY 10010-1710. Months of issue are March, June, September, and December. Periodicals postage paid at New York, NY and additional mailing offices. Subscription price per year is, $163.00 (US individuals), $557.00 (US institutions), $275.00 (international individuals), $680.00 (international institutions), $231.00 (Canadian individuals), $680.00 (Canadian institutions), $100.00 (US and Canadian students), and $135.00 (international students). To receive student/resident rate, orders must be accompanied by name of affiliated institution, date of term, and the signature of program/residency coordinator on institution letterhead. Orders will be billed at individual rate until proof of status is received. Foreign air speed delivery is included in all *Clinics* subscription prices. All prices are subject to change without notice. **POSTMASTER:** Send address changes to *Nursing Clinics*, Elsevier Health Sciences Division, Subscription Customer Service, 3251 Riverport Lane, Maryland Heights, MO 63043. **Customer Service: Telephone: 1-800-654-2452** (U.S. and Canada); **1-314-447-8871 (outside U.S. and Canada). Fax: 1-314-447-8029. E-mail: journalscustomerservice-usa@ elsevier.com** (for print support) and **journalsonlinesupport-usa@elsevier.com** (for online support).

*Nursing Clinics of North America* is covered in *EMBASE/Excerpta Medica, MEDLINE/PubMed (Index Medicus), Social Sciences Citation Index, Current Contents, ASCA, Cumulative Index to Nursing, RNdex Top 100,* and Allied Health Literature and International Nursing Index (INI).

# Contributors

## CONSULTING EDITOR

**BENJAMIN SMALLHEER, PhD, RN, ACNP-BC, FNP-BC, CCRN, CNE, FAANP**
Assistant Dean, Master of Science in Nursing Program, Associate Professor, Duke University School of Nursing, Durham, North Carolina

## EDITOR

**BRENT MACWILLIAMS, PhD, MSN, RN, APNP, ANP-BC**
Associate Professor, University of Wisconsin Oshkosh, College of Nursing, Oshkosh, Wisconsin

## AUTHORS

**CURRY JOSEPH BORDELON, DNP, MBA, NNP-BC, CNE**
The University of Alabama at Birmingham School of Nursing, Birmingham, Alabama

**CANDACE W. BURTON, PhD, RN, AFN-BC, FNAP**
Associate Professor, University of Nevada Las Vegas School of Nursing, Las Vegas, Nevada

**KATHLEEN M. ELERTSON, DNP, APNP, CPNP-PC, FNP-BC**
Associate Professor, University of Wisconsin Oshkosh, College of Nursing, Oshkosh, Wisconsin

**HEATHER M. ENGLUND, PhD, DNP, APNP, FNP-BC, CNE**
Associate Professor, University of Wisconsin Oshkosh, College of Nursing, Oshkosh, Wisconsin

**JULIAN L. GALLEGOS, PhD, MBA, FNP-BC, CNL, FAUNA**
Clinical Associate Professor, Purdue University, School of Nursing, West Lafayette, Indiana

**VERNON M. LANGFORD, DNP, APRN, FNP-C**
Citrus State Healthcare Consultants, PLLC, Altamonte Springs, Florida

**BRENT MACWILLIAMS, PhD, MSN, RN, APNP, ANP-BC**
Associate Professor, University of Wisconsin Oshkosh, College of Nursing, Oshkosh, Wisconsin; Associate Professor, University of Wisconsin Oshkosh, College of Nursing, Clintonville, Wisconsin

**ERIN MCARTHUR, BA, MA**
University of Wisconsin Oshkosh, College of Nursing, Oshkosh, Wisconsin

**LINDSAY L. MORGAN, DNP, APNP, FNP-BC**
Assistant Professor, University of Wisconsin Oshkosh, College of Nursing, Oshkosh, Wisconsin

**JASON MOTT, PhD, RN**
Prelicensure Program Director/Assistant Dean, University of Wisconsin Oshkosh, College of Nursing, Oshkosh, Wisconsin

**MELISSA D. PINTO, PhD, RN, FAAN**
Associate Professor, University of California, Irvine, Sue and Bill Gross School of Nursing, Irvine, California

**BLAKE K. SMITH, BSN, MSN, BS, RN**
Immediate Past President, Board of Directors, American Association for Men in Nursing, Wisconsin Rapids, Wisconsin; Clinical Documentation Sr. Analyst, Enterprise Applications, Nebraska Medicine, Accelerated Program Student Success Coach, School of Nursing, Nebraska Methodist College, Omaha, Nebraska

**JOACHIM G. VOSS, PhD, RN, ACRN, FAAN**
Professor, Case Western Reserve University, Frances Payne Bolton School of Nursing, Health Education Campus, Cleveland, Ohio

**MICHAEL WARD, MSN, APRN, AGACNP-BC**
Co-Owner, Founder and Chief Clinical Officer, Next Level TRT, LLC, Critical Care Nurse Practitioner, Cardiovascular ICU, Medical ICU, Texas Health Huguley Hospital, Burleson, Texas

# Contents

> Erectile dysfunction is a health condition that many men face in the United States. Nurses are primed to help men break the stigma; assess, manage, and treat the underlying factors; and educate men and their partner(s) regarding their health condition. Together they can work toward ensuring the patient maintains their sexual health and quality of life throughout their lifespan.

> In recent decades, much attention has been placed on reducing health disparities that have plagued the lesbian, gay, bisexual, transgender, and queer or questioning community. Significant health disparities continue to exist compared with the heterosexual population. Sexual minorities tend to experience higher rates of acute and chronic conditions than the general population. Sexual minorities are more likely to delay seeking medical care and are less likely to lack a consistent source for health care. A provider's failure to recognize and a person's lack of disclosure prevent vital discussions about human immunodeficiency virus risk, hormone therapy, cancer risk, hepatitis, and sexual health.

> Men are taking on a caregiving role more often in society. This article will explore the history of men in the caregiving role, how men provide care and practical strategies on how to assist men who find themselves in the caregiving role.

Suicide and the risk factors associated with it have been researched with increasing interest over the last 5 decades with respect to socioeconomic status, age, geographic location, and ethnic background. There has been less focus related to the risk factors specific to gender and how to incorporate clinical screening and interventions to reduce the mortality of suicide in males. With men accounting for a disproportionate number of deaths from suicide in the United States and worldwide, how gender could impact suicidal behavior and ideations remains a topic understudied and with great potential for significant improvement in clinical recognition and treatment.

Over the last 3 decades, there has been an increased interest in testosterone replacement therapy. This trend is a result of an aging population, endocrine disruptors in our foods and environment and rising obesity rates. In addition, there has been a surge in Men's Health clinics and online direct-to-consumer Web sites, making testosterone replacement therapy much more readily accessible. As more men seek to increase their testosterone levels, more long-term random control studies are needed to gain better insight into testosterone optimization to support the anecdotal observation commonly experienced in the practice setting.

The review critically analyzes the social determinants of health (SDOH) variables in the current literature of patients with post-acute sequelae (PASC) of COVID-19 in the United States. Race, gender, and age were discussed as well as health outcomes, severity of illness, and phenotypes of long-COVID. Most research was retrospectively with samples that had access to health insurance, which did not capture populations with poor or no access to health care. More research is needed that directly addresses the impact on SDOH on PASC. The current literature is sparse and provides little actionable information.

Although telehealth seems to be an emerging technological marvel, it has been used in some way for many years now. Moreover, although the coronavirus disease 2019 pandemic wreaked horrific and tragic havoc around the world, it brought with it a new era of patient-centered care that forced many reluctant providers to adopt its use. With newer technologies at our fingertips and on the horizon and an increased number of qualified men's health specialists coming to the fore, men's telehealth will increasingly continue to provide a viable option for men seeking care and treatment.

Unmet holistic needs of various cancer populations, with examples including prostate, bladder, gynecologic, kidney, penile, breast, and colorectal, along with holistic impacts of cancer on older adults, have been defined by a growing number of systematic reviews. Unfortunately, there continues to be a lack of clinical insight into the unique needs of younger men with testicular cancer. Survival rate based on low mortality rates and good prognosis if early detection and treatment implementation grows the number of men who need support as long-term survivors with an average life expectancy of approximately 30 to 50 years after treatment. Providers and clinicians need to approach testicular cancer survivors with the tools and strategies that meet these unmet needs for navigation from diagnosis through survivorship. When strategies of specific resources and education are implemented based on the unique needs of these individuals, positive outcomes and increased health care-related quality of life will be prevalent.

According to the World Health Organization, heart disease is the leading cause of death worldwide, accounting for approximately 17.9 million deaths annually. Although both men and women experience heart disease, there are notable differences in pathophysiology, evaluation, and pharmacologic management related to biological sex and gender. Men are more likely to develop heart disease at younger ages with more severe presentations. Women usually develop heart disease later in life and have more subtle symptoms, including microvascular involvement. It is essential that providers are aware of gender disparities, social determinants, and modifiable risk factors in prevention of heart disease.

All people face end of life as the final health outcome. When a person's health focus shifts from quantity to quality of life, palliative care comes into view. Clinicians serving patients across the health care spectrum must be aware of the nature and efficacy of palliative and hospice care, indications for referral to services, and current best practices. Creating an end-of-life trajectory requires an individualized and global personal plan, which palliative and hospice care can provide. Gender-specific care that includes gender minorities provides special and unique challenges to those seeking palliative and hospice care.

While numbers of men in the nursing profession have slowly increased, men in female-dominated specialty areas have not changed. Male nurses and nursing students encounter gender bias and discrimination in certain specialty nursing environments. This has implications for the quality of care provided, parental engagement, and job satisfaction. By diversifying the nursing workforce, there is a potential to enhance patient comfort, improve satisfaction, and promote a more inclusive, creative, and patient-focused health care environment.

Hormone therapy is a common treatment method for adult males, females, and transgender and gender-diverse individuals. Both men, women, and transgender and gender-diverse people may use hormone therapy at some point in their lives. There are notable differences and similarities in risk factors related to hormone therapy use based on genetics, sex, gender, personal history, and the type of hormone therapy used. Provider awareness in gender-inclusive hormone therapy management with the consideration of nonmodifiable and modifiable risk factors, prevention of complications, and monitoring parameters is essential in clinical practice.

# NURSING CLINICS

**SERIES OF RELATED INTEREST**

*Advances in Family Practice Nursing*
*www.advancesinfamilypracticenursing.com*

**THE CLINICS ARE AVAILABLE ONLINE!**
Access your subscription at:
www.theclinics.com

# Foreword

# Men's Health and Men in Health Care

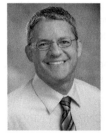

Benjamin Smallheer, PhD, RN, ACNP-BC, FNP-BC, CCRN, CNE, FAANP
*Consulting Editor*

The phrase "nursing care" immediately brings an image to many people's minds. It may be a mental image of Florence Nightingale serving the soldiers of the Crimean War: her long dress, working long shifts by candlelight, advocating for soldiers to have clean air and fresh linens. Often, the next thought may be of our iconic nursing leaders through time, such as Clara Barton, Loretta Ford, and maybe…just may-be…Luther Christman and Walt Whitman (yes, Walt Whitman was a nurse!!!). Finally, nursing care may be identified along the lines of disease processes and care settings: cardiovascular nursing, critical care nursing, community health, and population health nursing. But what about nursing across the sex and gender spectrum? The concepts of social determinates of health, health inequities, and social injustices are strongly being advocated for within nursing. Our marginalized populations are coming into our central focus to improve health outcomes and decrease the health care gap. One of these marginalized and underrepresented areas of health care is men's health.

The statistics associated with men's health from the Centers of Disease Control and Prevention[1,2] are staggering.

For men aged 18 years of age or over,[1,2]

- 13.2% report currently smoking cigarettes
- 40.5% struggle with obesity
- 51.9% have been diagnosed with hypertension
- Prostate cancer is the number 2 cause of cancer-related deaths

When surveyed,[3]

- 38% of men are concerned about urologic cancers
- 32% are concerned about sexual health

Nurs Clin N Am 58 (2023) xi–xii
https://doi.org/10.1016/j.cnur.2023.07.006
0029-6465/23/© 2023 Published by Elsevier Inc.

- Up to 77% of men do not know their family health history of men's health issues
- 55% of men report not getting regular health screenings

In this issue, we aim to move the needle and draw much needed attention to health promotion and disease prevention within men's health. Together, the authors present a dynamic variety of gender-specific topics, such as heart disease prevention within the male gender, LBGTQI+ health disparities, risk factors for suicide in men, testicular cancer, testosterone and gender-specific hormone replacement, and erectile dysfunction. The authors even go one step farthere to providing insight and perspective into the roles of the male caregiver, telehealth strategies within men's health, men in female-dominated nursing specialties, and men and gender-specific roles within hospice and palliative care.

It is our goal, through the planning and production of this issue of *Nursing Clinics of North America*, to create a resource on Men's Health and Men in Health Care for providers across the globe.

Benjamin Smallheer, PhD, RN, ACNP-BC, FNP-BC, CCRN, CNE, FAANP
Assistant Dean
Master of Science in Nursing Program
Associate Professor
School of Nursing
Duke University
307 Trent Drive, Box 3322, Office 3117
Durham, NC 27710, USA

*E-mail address:*
benjamin.smallheer@duke.edu

**REFERENCES**

1. National Center for Health Statistics (June 30, 2023). Men's health. Available at: https://www.cdc.gov/nchs/fastats/mens-health.htm. Accessed July 21, 2023.
2. Centers for Disease Control and Prevention (June 8, 2023). Prostate cancer statistics. Available at: https://www.cdc.gov/cancer/prostate/statistics/index.htm. Accessed July 21, 2023.
3. Cleveland Clinic (September 7, 2022). Cleveland Clinic survey reveals men's top health concerns as they age. Available at: https://newsroom.clevelandclinic.org/2022/09/07/cleveland-clinic-survey-reveals-mens-top-health-concerns-as-they-age/. Accessed July 21, 2023.

# Preface

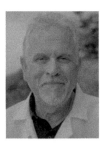

Brent MacWilliams, PhD, MSN, RN, APNP, ANP-BC
*Editor*

Men's health and disease prevention are typically limited to male-specific health viewed with a binary gender lens. In this issue of *Nursing Clinics of North America*, we explore more inclusive perspectives regarding gender in the context of a variety of issues and disorders to offer new clinical insights.

The authors offer a vision for gender as a nonbinary continuum to reimage men's health that is clinically current and more inclusive. The reimaging provides nurses, advanced practice nurses, physicians, and other health care providers with new insights into the most recent literature regarding men's health. The authors cover long-haul COVID-19 symptoms in diverse populations, heart disease prevention and gender, health disparities in the LBGTQI+ community, male caregiving, risk factors for suicide in men, testicular cancer—current best practice, low testosterone—current best practice, men's health as a telehealth strategy, erectile dysfunction: a holistic review, hospice, and palliative care—men and gender-specific roles, gender-specific hormone replacement therapies, and men in female-dominated nursing specialties.

The goal was to create a catalog of evidence-based articles to update health care providers on a unique population and the challenges for an underrepresented population providing that health care.

Brent MacWilliams, PhD, MSN, RN, APNP, ANP-BC
University of Wisconsin–
Oshkosh College of Nursing
800 Algoma Boulevard
Oshkosh, WI 54901, USA

*E-mail address:*
macwillb@uwosh.edu

# In Memoriam

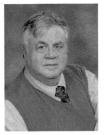

Stephen D. Krau, PhD, RN, CNE

Dr Stephen D. Krau, former Consulting Editor for the *Nursing Clinics of North America*, passed away on August 18, 2023.

For a decade, Dr Krau served as the Consulting Editor, providing important oversight and guidance on our content. He ensured that our issues and articles had high utility among bedside nurses, with a focus on patient assessment, expected outcomes, interventions, rationale, and evaluation, with an eye on evidentiary support. He also had the foresight to identify gaps in coverage of topics that were clinically useful for nurses but weren't readily available in the literature. Dr Krau seemed to have his pulse on what was important currently and the vision to see what would be essential in the future. His passion for nursing was evident in the composition of his forewords for each issue, which were engaging and full of insights. One of his forewords has been highly cited and continues to be even 6 years later: "The Difference Between Palliative Care and End of Life Care: More than Semantics." He eloquently defines the similarities and differences of palliative care, end-of-life care, and hospice care and describes how they intertwine. He said, "The differences are very explicit and important as decisions and plans are made for patients and their significant others."

Our editorial and production staff is so deeply saddened by his passing. It was indeed our privilege to work with him in every pleasant interaction. Even when he had to deliver bad news or discuss a negative situation, he did it with such thoughtfulness and compassion. We will miss our collaborations with him and his positive outlook.

We feel so very lucky and honored to have worked with him. Anyone who ever read an article from *Nursing Clinics of North America* was touched by his commitment to educating and supporting nurses. He will be greatly missed.

Kerry Holland
Senior Editor
*Nursing Clinics of North America*
Elsevier Inc
1600 JFK Blvd
Philadelphia, PA 19103

Nurs Clin N Am 58 (2023) xv
https://doi.org/10.1016/j.cnur.2023.09.001
0029-6465/23/© 2023 Published by Elsevier Inc.

nursing.theclinics.com

# Erectile Dysfunction
## Current Best Practices

Julian L. Gallegos, PhD, MBA, FNP-BC, CNL, FAUNA

### KEYWORDS

- Erectile dysfunction • Men's health • Sexual health

### KEY POINTS

- Erectile dysfunction in men is common, especially after the age of 40 years.
- Underlying health conditions predispose men to erectile dysfunction.
- Dispelling the stigma and having open conversations about erectile dysfunction with men is essential in addressing treatment and management.
- There are several pharmacologic and nonpharmacological treatments available to treat erectile dysfunction.
- Nurses play a vital role in treating and managing erectile dysfunction in men.

## INTRODUCTION

Sexual health is an important aspect of an individual's life. As men move through the phases of aging, sexuality and sex can take on different forms. For many men, their sexuality is defined by their ability to perform in the proverbial bedroom, which includes their ability to obtain erections to have sexual relations with their partner. Erections for men are an essential aspect of their sexual identity regardless of sexual orientation. When obtaining or maintaining erections becomes difficult, men often face multiple complex emotions. They often choose not to disclose this issue to anyone, including their health care provider, due to embarrassment or feeling inferior.

Erectile dysfunction (ED) is a condition in which a male cannot get or keep an erection firm enough for satisfactory sexual intercourse.[1–4] ED can be short term or long term. An individual is considered to have ED when[1,3,4]

- The individual can obtain erections sometimes, but not every time they want to have sex.
- The individual can obtain erections, but the erection does not last long enough for fulfilling or satisfactory sex.
- The individual is unable to get an erection at any time.

---

Purdue University, Johnson Hall, Room 256A, 502 North University Street, West Lafayette, IN 47907, USA
*E-mail address:* jlgalleg@purdue.edu

Nurs Clin N Am 58 (2023) 483–493
https://doi.org/10.1016/j.cnur.2023.06.001
0029-6465/23/© 2023 Elsevier Inc. All rights reserved.

ED is a common problem among men in the United States (US). The prevalence of ED increases with age, with the estimates suggesting that it affects around 50% of men over the age of 40 years.[1,5,6] The National Institutes of Health estimate that ED affects about 18 million men in the US alone.[5] The prevalence of ED is also higher among those who have certain health conditions such as diabetes, hypertension, and cardiovascular disease.[1,5,7,8] ED is not a normal part of aging and can be treated by the individual consulting with a health care provider and addressing the underlying medical conditions predisposing them to the symptoms.[2,6]

Because of the prevalence of ED in the US, nurses must become aware of the implications associated with ED and learn how to help treat men affected by this condition. Nurses maintain the skills and expertise to readily address the disorder by understanding the phenomena associated with this health condition.

### Stigma of ED

Due to the stigma often associated with the condition, ED can be a sensitive and challenging subject for many men. The stigma of ED can make it difficult for men to seek help and treatment, ultimately leading to a decline in their sexual quality of life. A significant cause for the stigma associated with ED is the cultural perception of masculinity and the belief that men should always be able to perform sexually.[9-11] This preconceived notion can make it challenging for men to admit to themselves and others that they are experiencing ED, as they may feel it is a sign of weakness or emasculation.[9-11] Another reason for the stigma surrounding ED is the lack of education and understanding regarding the condition. Many believe ED is simply a natural part of aging that cannot be treated; however, this is not necessarily true because ED can have multiple underlying causes that can be treated.

Furthermore, the stigma of ED can make it difficult for men to talk to their health care provider about their condition and the symptoms they are experiencing. They often feel embarrassed or ashamed to discuss the subject, and health care providers may not always discuss it during routine health visits.[9-11] Because of the stigmas associated with ED, there can be delays in seeking treatment, which can negatively impact the sexual health and quality of life of those affected by ED. As a health care provider, breaking down this stigmatization by creating more awareness and understanding of the condition is vital. Health care providers must encourage men to trust them to talk about ED if they are experiencing symptoms and to educate them that ED is a common condition that can be treated.

Men may be sensitive in discussing ED for several reasons that health care providers must be aware of. Some of these reasons may include the following.[9-11]

- Embarrassment: ED can be a sensitive and personal topic, and some men may feel embarrassed or ashamed about their condition, making it difficult to discuss it openly.
- Stigma: There may be a societal stigma attached to ED, with men feeling it is a sign of weakness or lack of masculinity. This can make it difficult for men to talk about their condition, even with a health care provider.
- Fear of rejection: Men with ED may fear rejection from their partners and may be hesitant to discuss the condition with them out of fear that it will negatively impact their relationship.
- Fear of not having a solution: Some men may fear that there is no solution to their ED and that discussing it with a health care provider will be futile.
- Lack of knowledge: Some men may not be aware of the various treatment options available for ED or may not understand the underlying causes of their

condition. This can make it difficult for them to discuss it with a health care provider.

### Psychological Effects of ED

Due to the stigma associated with ED, many men suffer psychological effects related to ED. If the individual was not already suffering from underlying psychological issues causing the ED, some of the common psychological effects that a health care provider must be aware of with men affected by ED are listed here.[9,12]

- Low self-esteem: Men with ED may feel inadequate, leading to low self-esteem and embarrassment.
- Depression: ED can cause feelings of sadness, hopelessness, and worthlessness, leading to depression.
- Relationship problems: ED can strain relationships and cause both partners frustration, anger, or resentment.
- Reduces sexual desire: ED can cause a lack of sexual desire, which can have a negative impact on a man's overall quality of life.

For a health care provider, it is crucial to make sure that men affected by ED deduce that these feelings are normal and understandable. Health care providers must know that many effective ED treatments are available, including lifestyle changes, medications, and therapy. Counseling and therapy can help men with ED cope with the psychological effects of the condition. Health care providers must address the psychological effects of ED and ensure that men understand that ED is not a sign of weakness or failure.

### Effects of Pornography on ED

The effects of pornography on ED are a topic of ongoing research and debate. Some studies suggest that excessive use of pornography can lead to ED, while others have found no significant link between the two.[13] One theory is that viewing pornography can lead to desensitization to real-life sexual partners, making it difficult for men to become aroused to maintain an erection during sexual activity.[13] In addition, some men may develop unrealistic expectations about sexual performance and physical appearance, contributing to anxiety and self-consciousness during sexual encounters.[13]

On the other hand, some experts suggest that moderate use of pornography can positively affect sexual function by improving sexual desire and sexual satisfaction. It is important to note that further research is needed to fully understand the relationship between pornography and ED, and the effects may vary from person to person.

### Sexual Preference and ED

Sexual preference, orientation, and ED are separate issues that sometimes intersect. ED can affect men, regardless of sexual preference or orientation, and men who identify as gay, bisexual, or heterosexual can all experience ED. Literature suggests that men who identify as gay or bisexual may be at higher risk of ED due to factors such as increased stress and anxiety related to societal stigmatization and discrimination.[14,15] Furthermore, men who have sex with men may have a higher risk of certain sexually transmitted infections that can contribute to developing ED.[14,15]

Regarding sexual preference and orientation, it is crucial for health care providers to know that ED is a medical condition that can be treated regardless of sexual orientation or preference. Health care providers should attune to the sensitive and unique needs of their patients. Gay and bisexual men often have unique concerns that need support from health care providers in providing information and support in helping manage ED and other sexual health concerns not experienced by their heterosexual counterparts.[14,15]

### Race and ED

Race may play a role in the rates of ED, as some studies have found that certain racial and ethnic groups have a higher prevalence of ED than others. However, it is essential to note that these studies are inconclusive, and more research is needed to understand the relationship between race and ED fully. Some studies have found that African American men may have a higher prevalence of ED than White or Hispanic men.[16–18] This may be attributed to a higher prevalence of risk factors associated with ED, such as hypertension and diabetes, in this population. Other studies have found that Hispanic men may have a lower prevalence of ED than non-Hispanic White men.[16,18] This may be due to differences in lifestyle and cultural practices, such as diet and physical activity levels. It is also important to note that other factors, such as socioeconomic status, access to health care, and education, also play a role in the prevalence of ED.

### Age and ED

Although age is not a direct cause of ED, underlying medical conditions that affect men as they age are most likely to occur predominantly in men older than 40 years. As men age, their risk for certain health conditions that contribute to ED, such as hypertension, diabetes, and heart disease, increases. These conditions lead to a change in the blood vessels through a process of endothelial dysfunction affecting the ability of nitric oxide to make the necessary changes within the blood vessels to allow blood to flow to the penis during arousal, thus causing ED.[1,2,6]

Furthermore, after the age of 40 years, men lose approximately 1% of total testosterone yearly.[2] This decline in testosterone can lead to decreased sexual desire and resultant ED.[2] Aging can also bring psychological changes contributing to ED, such as stress, anxiety, and depression.[6] Despite ED not being related to aging, it is essential that health care providers routinely screen older men for ED and other sexual health concerns and provide appropriate care and treatment. This can improve their sexual health and overall quality of life.

### Causes of ED

ED is a complex condition with multiple causes. The pathophysiology of ED involves a complex interplay of physiologic, psychological, and lifestyle factors that can interfere with the normal physiologic processes that result in an erection. Physiologically, an erection occurs when the spongy tissue in the penis fills with blood, causing it to become stiff and erect. This process is controlled by the nervous system and involves the release of nitric oxide, a chemical that relaxes the blood vessels in the penis and allows blood to flow into the penis.[4,19–21]

The most common causes of ED include vascular problems, such as atherosclerosis or hypertension; neurologic problems, such as nerve damage from diabetes or spinal cord injuries; hormonal imbalances, such as low testosterone levels; and psychological problems, such as stress or anxiety.[4,19–21] Vascular issues can lead to ED by causing a decrease in blood flow to the penis, making it difficult to achieve or maintain an erection. Neurologic problems can cause ED by disrupting the nerve signals necessary for an erection. Hormonal imbalances can also cause ED by disrupting the balance of hormones essential for sexual function. Psychological problems can cause ED by causing anxiety disorders or stress, making it difficult to relax and become sexually aroused.

In most cases, ED is caused by a combination of factors. The underlying pathophysiology of ED involves the inability of the penile vessels to dilate and fill with blood to achieve and maintain an erection. This can be due to structural changes in the vessels, dysfunction of the smooth muscle cells, or a combination of both. Diagnosis of ED typically begins with a thorough history and physical examination and may include further testing such as blood tests, psychological evaluation, nocturnal tumescence, and rigidity testing.[3,7,21–23]

Often ED is accompanied by concomitant sexual disorders. Health care providers must be aware of these disorders and evaluate them with ED. Some of the most common sexual conditions that accompany ED include[4,19–21]

- Premature ejaculation: This is a condition in which a man ejaculates earlier than he or his partner would like. It can be a separate disorder or happen in conjunction with ED.
- Delayed ejaculation: This is a condition in which a man takes a longer time to ejaculate than he or his partner would like. It can be a separate disorder or happen in conjunction with ED.
- Low libido: Also known as hypoactive sexual desire disorder, a condition in which a man has reduced interest in sexual activity.
- Anorgasmia: This is the inability to achieve orgasm; it can be a separate disorder or happen in conjunction with ED.
- Peyronie's disease: This is a condition in which scar tissue forms inside the penis, causing it to bend or curve during an erection.
- Male hypogonadism: This is a condition in which the body does not produce enough testosterone, which can lead to a decreased sex drive and ED.

Awareness by the health care provider of these potential underlying and concomitant health conditions contributing to or causing ED is essential in ensuring that the individual's care is maximized through a holistic approach to their condition.

### Assessing for ED

ED assessment involves a thorough medical history, physical examination, and diagnostic tests. During the medical history, the health care provider should ask about the patient's symptoms, including the duration and severity of ED, and any other related symptoms, such as premature ejaculation, low libido, and difficulty achieving orgasm. The health care provider should also ask about any medical conditions, medications, and lifestyle factors contributing to ED.[4,19,20]

When bringing up the topic of ED in men during a health visit, the clinician must be sensitive, empathetic, and nonjudgmental. Some suggestions for the clinician in approaching the visit include[4,19,20,22]

- Use open-ended questions: Ask the patient if he has any concerns or questions about his sexual health, which can help initiate the conversation in a nonthreatening way.
- Provide privacy: Make sure the patient is in a private room, and there are no interruptions during the conversation and examination.
- Provide education: Explain that ED is a common condition affecting many men and that various treatment options are available.
- Address any underlying health conditions: Ask the patient if he has any underlying health conditions, such as diabetes, hypertension, or cardiovascular disease, which can contribute to ED.

- Encourage the patient to speak freely: Let him know that he must be honest about his symptoms and concerns and that there is no shame in discussing ED.
- Provide resources: Let the patient know that various resources are available to help him, such as brochures, websites, or support groups.

The physical examination should include a genital and prostate examination. The health care provider should assess for signs of decreased blood flow to the penis, such as diminished penile sensation. Diagnostic tests that may be used to evaluate for ED include[4,19,20,22]

- Blood test: to assess for conditions such as diabetes, low testosterone levels, and high cholesterol
- Psychological evaluation: to assess for psychological factors that may contribute to ED
- Nocturnal penile tumescence and rigidity testing: to evaluate the ability of the patient to achieve an erection during sleep
- Duplex ultrasound: to assess blood flow to the penis
- Penile angiogram: to assess blood vessels in the penis
- Corpus cavernosometry and cavernosograpy: to evaluate the structure and function of the blood vessels in the penis.

The clinician should take a systematic approach to the diagnosis of ED by using a comprehensive approach for evaluation that considers not only the physical symptoms but also the psychological, relational, and lifestyle factors that may contribute to ED.

### Pharmacologic Treatment of ED

Pharmacologic treatments for ED offer several benefits for men experiencing this condition. Medications for ED have been extensively studied and proven effective in improving erections and sexual function.[4,20,23] These medications increase blood flow to the penis, making it easier to achieve and maintain an erection.[4,20,23] They are also generally safe when used as directed and under the guidance of a health care provider, with few serious side effects. Pharmacologic treatments for ED are also convenient, as they can be taken orally and used as needed without extensive preparation or planning. Restoring sexual function can significantly impact a man's quality of life, relationships, and overall well-being.

Several medications are commonly used to treat ED. These include[4,20,23,24]

- Phosphodiesterase type 5 (PDE5) inhibitors: These medications work by increasing blood flow to the penis. These medications are typically available in oral form and are taken at least 1 hour before intercourse. During penile erections, cyclic guanosine monophosphate (cGMP) is metabolized through the PDE5 enzyme and cannot exert its downstream erectile effects. PDE5 inhibitors are selective, competitive, and reversible, generally decreasing cGMP metabolism and ultimately leading to the successful attainment and maintenance of an erection.[25] Examples of PDE5s include sildenafil, tadalafil, and vardenafil.
- Alprostadil: This medication can be injected into the penis or the urethra as a pellet. It works by increasing blood flow to the penis.
- Testosterone replacement therapy (TRT): Low testosterone levels can lead to ED; TRT may be prescribed for men with low testosterone levels. Testosterone affects nitric oxide production and PDE5 expression in the corpus cavernosum, which helps preserve muscle contractility by regulating contraction and relaxation and supports the structure of the corpus cavernosum.[26]

These medications may not be suitable for every individual. The health care provider must be aware of potential side effects. Common side effects of these types of medications include[4,19,23]

- Headache
- Nasal congestion
- Flushing
- Hypotension
- Altered colored vision.

### Nonpharmacological Treatment of ED

Along with pharmacologic treatments for ED, there are nonpharmacological treatments that men can try to assist in reducing or eliminating the incidence of ED. The nonpharmacological treatments for ED include[24,27]

- Behavioral therapy: This can help address any underlying psychological or emotional issues contributing to ED.
- Lifestyle changes: Quitting smoking, exercising regularly, and eating a healthy diet can improve blood flow and overall health, which can, in turn, improve ED symptoms.
- Penile pumps: A vacuum erection device can create an erection by drawing blood into the penis.
- Penile implants: A surgical option for men who do not respond to other treatments, penile implants involve the placement of a device into the penis that allows for an erection.
- Acupuncture: Some studies have suggested that acupuncture may be effective in improving ED symptoms although more research is needed to confirm this.
- Counseling or sex therapy: This can assist men and their partners in better understanding and coping with ED and can also help address any relationship issues contributing to the problem.

Although nonpharmacological treatments for ED can be effective, there are potential downsides to consider. Some nonpharmacological treatments, such as vacuum devices and penile implants, can be expensive and not covered by insurance. Psychological counseling may also be costly and may require ongoing sessions. In addition, some nonpharmacological treatments may not be suitable for everyone, and it is essential to talk to a health care provider to determine the best treatment approach. There may also be side effects or complications associated with some treatments, such as discomfort or infection from a penile implant. Furthermore, some nonpharmacological treatments may require time and effort to see results, and some men may prefer the convenience of medication.[27] It is important to weigh the potential benefits and drawbacks of nonpharmacological treatments before deciding on a treatment approach for ED.

### Partner Participation in Treatment of ED

Partner participation in the treatment of ED is vital because ED has an impact on both partners. Involving the partner in the treatment process can help to improve communication and understanding about the condition and can help to reduce feelings of stress, anxiety, and frustration.[9,28,29]

There are several ways a partner can participate in the treatment of ED.[9,28]

- Support: Partners can provide emotional support to their loved ones by listening, being patient, and understanding the impact of ED on their relationship.

- Lifestyle changes: Partners can support their loved ones by changing their lifestyles, such as eating a healthy diet and exercising together.
- Therapy: Partners can participate in couples therapy or sex therapy to improve communication and intimacy.
- Medication and treatment: Partners can help remind the patient to take their medication and keep track of the treatment schedule.
- Encouragement: Partners can encourage their loved on to seek help and to talk to a health care provider about their condition.

ED is not just a man's issue but a couple's issue. A partner's participation in treatment can help to improve the outcome for the patient and the relationship.

### Nurse's Role in the Management of ED

Nurses are primed to help men with ED. Nurses at all educational levels can play a significant role. Their responsibilities in helping manage ED in men include[3,7,23,30]

- Assessment: Nurses can perform a thorough physical examination and take a detailed medical history to determine the underlying causes of ED.
- Diagnosis: Nurse practitioners (NPs) can diagnose ED by considering the patient's symptoms, medical history, and examination results.
- Treatment: NPs can prescribe medications such as PDE5s to treat ED. They can also recommend lifestyle changes such as diet and exercise to improve overall health.
- Follow-up care: Nurses can monitor the patient's response to treatment, and NPs can adjust the medications as needed. Nurses can also provide patients with education and support to help them manage their condition.
- Referral: If necessary, NPs can refer patients to specialists such as urologists or sex therapists to receive further evaluation and treatment.

Furthermore, nurses can help break the stigma associated with ED, playing a pivotal role in this process. Some ways that a nurse can help break the stigma for men with ED include[3,7,23,30,31]

- Education: Nurses can educate men about the causes and risk factors for ED and help them understand that it is not a sign of weakness or failure.
- Normalizing the conversation: Nurses can talk openly and comfortably about ED with the patient and make sure that men understand that it is a common condition many men experience.
- Providing accurate information: Nurses can provide accurate information about ED and the available treatments, which can help to reduce fear, anxiety, and embarrassment.
- Encouraging patients to seek help: Nurses can encourage men to seek help for ED and talk to their partners about the condition.
- Collaboration with other health care providers: Nurses can work with other health care providers, such as urologists, sex therapists, and mental health professionals, to provide comprehensive care for men with ED.
- Breaking the language barriers: Nurses should ensure their patients understand the information provided, especially those whose primary language is not English. This can be done by using simple language, providing translated materials, and having a translator available to discuss their health concern.

Overall, nurses play an essential role in managing ED in men and can help break the stigma associated with the health condition through their diverse range of skills and expertise. By providing patient education, counseling, and medication management services, nurses can help improve the quality of life for patients affected by this condition and contribute to the overall success of ED treatment plans.

## SUMMARY

Nurses must become aware of ED because it is a common condition that can significantly affect men's physical and emotional health. Nurses play a vital role in assessing and managing patients with ED, including educating them about the causes and treatment options available. Nurses can help patients overcome this condition's stigma by being knowledgeable about ED and empowering them to seek the care they need.

ED is often a symptom of underlying conditions such as cardiovascular disease, diabetes, and hypertension. Nurses familiar with ED can recognize this connection and refer patients for further evaluation and treatment. ED can be an early warning sign of these conditions in some cases, allowing for earlier diagnosis and intervention to improve outcomes. Nurses can work collaboratively with other health care providers to manage these underlying conditions, which can, in turn, improve ED symptoms and the overall quality of life for patients.

Furthermore, ED can be a source of emotional distress and relationship issues for men and their partners. Nurses knowledgeable about ED can provide counseling and support to patients and their partners, helping them cope with the psychological impact of this condition. By being compassionate and nonjudgmental, nurses can create a safe and supportive environment for patients to discuss their concerns and seek the care they need.

In conclusion, ED is a common condition that can significantly impact men's physical and emotional health. Nurses knowledgeable about ED can play a crucial role in assessing and managing patients with this condition, identifying underlying medical conditions, and providing emotional support to patients and their partners. By being aware of ED and its implications, nurses can help improve outcomes and quality of life for patients affected by this condition.

## DISCLOSURE

The author has nothing to disclose.

## REFERENCES

1. Allen MS, Walter EE. Erectile dysfunction: an umbrella review of meta-analyses of risk-factors, treatment, and prevalence outcomes. Journal of Sexual Medicine 2019;16(4):531–41.
2. Aleksandra R, Aleksandra S, Iwona R. Erectile Dysfunction in Relation to Metabolic Disorders and the Concentration of Sex Hormones in Aging Men. Int J Environ Res Publ Health 2022;19(13):7576.
3. Lewis JH. The role of the NP in the diagnosis and management of erectile dysfunction. The Nurse Practitioner 2000;25(3):14–8.
4. Mirone V, Fusco F, Cirillo L, Napolitano L. Erectile Dysfunction: From Pathophysiology to Clinical Assessment. In: Bettocchi C, Busetto GM, Carrieri G, Cormio L, editors. Practical Clinical Andrology. Cham: Springer; 2023. https://doi.org/10.1007/978-3-031-11701-5_3.
5. National Institutes of Health. NIH Consensus Conference. Impotence. NIH consensus development panel on impotence. JAMA 1993;270:83–90.

6. Pellegrino F, Sjoberg DD, Tin AL, et al. Relationship Between Age, Comorbidity, and the Prevalence of Erectile Dysfunction. Eur Urol Focus 2023;9(1):162–7.

7. Steggall MJ. Clinical management of erectile dysfunction. International Journal of Urological Nursing 2011;5(2):52–8.

8. Thomas JA. Pharmacological aspects of erectile dysfunction. Jpn J Pharmacol 2002;89(2):101–12.

9. Dewitte M, Bettocchi C, Carvalho J, et al. A psychosocial approach to erectile dysfunction: position statements from the European Society of Sexual Medicine (ESSM). Sex Med 2021;9(6):100434–100434.

10. Foster S, Pomerantz A, Bell K, Carvallo M, et al. Victims of virility: Honor endorsement, stigma, and men's use of erectile dysfunction medication. Psychology of Men & Masculinities 2022;23(1):47.

11. Sharma A, Sharma RP. Erectile Dysfunction: The Male Stigma. Int J Surg 2019;5: 172–8.

12. Sheng Z. Psychological consequences of erectile dysfunction. Trends in Urology & Men's Health 2021;12(6):19–22.

13. Jacobs T, Geysemans B, Van Hal G, et al. Associations between online pornography consumption and sexual dysfunction in young men: multivariate analysis based on an international web-based survey. JMIR public health and surveillance 2021;7(10):e32542.

14. Barbonetti A, D'Andrea S, Cavallo F, et al. Erectile dysfunction and premature ejaculation in homosexual and heterosexual men: a systematic review and meta-analysis of comparative studies. J Sex Med 2019;16(5):624–32.

15. Fernandez-Crespo RE, Cordon-Galiano BH. Sexual dysfunction among men who have sex with men: a review article. Curr Urol Rep 2021;22:1–7.

16. Chen T, Shufeng L, Michael L, et al. Associations between Race and Erectile Dysfunction Treatment Patterns. Urology Practice 2022;9(5):423–30.

17. Cripps SM, Mattiske DM, Pask AJ. Erectile dysfunction in men on the rise: is there a link with endocrine disrupting chemicals? Sex Dev 2021;15(1–3):187–212.

18. Saigal CS, Wessells H, Pace J, et al. Predictors and prevalence of erectile dysfunction in a racially diverse population. Arch Intern Med 2006;166(2):207–12.

19. MacDonald SM, Burnett AL. Physiology of erection and pathophysiology of erectile dysfunction. Urologic Clinics 2021;48(4):513–25.

20. Trebatický B, Žitňanová I, Dvořáková M, et al. Role of oxidative stress, adiponectin and endoglin in the pathophysiology of erectile dysfunction in diabetic and non-diabetic men. Physiol Res 2019;68(4):623–31.

21. Wright LN, Moghalu OI, Das R, et al. Erectile dysfunction and treatment: An analysis of associated chronic health conditions. Urology 2021;157:148–54.

22. McMahon CG. Current diagnosis and management of erectile dysfunction. Med J Aust 2019;210(10):469–76.

23. Schreiber ML. Erectile Dysfunction. Medsurg Nursing 2019;28(5):327–30.

24. Krzastek SC, Bopp J, Smith RP, et al. Recent advances in the understanding and management of erectile dysfunction. F1000Research 2019;8.

25. Shamloul R, Ghanem H. Erectile dysfunction. Lancet 2013;381(9861):153–65.

26. Kataoka T, Kimura K. Testosterone and erectile function: a review of evidence from basic research. Sex Hormones in Neurodegenerative Processes and Diseases 2018;257–72.

27. Wassersug R, Wibowo E. Non-pharmacological and non-surgical strategies to promote sexual recovery for men with erectile dysfunction. Transl Androl Urol 2017;6(Suppl 5):S776.

28. Dorey G. Partner's perspective of erectile dysfunction: literature review. Br J Nurs 2001;10(3):187–95.
29. Green R, Kodish S. Discussing a sensitive topic: nurse practitioners and physician assistants' communication strategies in managing patients with erectile dysfunction. J Am Acad Nurse Pract 2009;21(12):698–705.
30. Albaugh JA, Kellogg-Spadt S. Sexuality and sexual health: The nurse's role and initial approach to patients. Urol Nurs 2003;23(3):227–8.
31. Al-Shaiji TF. Breaking the Ice of Erectile Dysfunction Taboo: A Focus on Clinician–Patient Communication. Journal of Patient Experience 2022;9. 23743735221077512.

# Minority Stress and Health Disparities in Lesbian, Gay, Bisexual, Transgender, and Queer or Questioning Adults

Heather M. Englund, PhD, DNP

## KEYWORDS

- Lesbian, gay, bisexual, transgender, and queer or questioning health
- Health disparities • Minority stress • LGBTQ curriculum • Medical education
- Nursing education

## KEY POINTS

- Despite growing attention being placed on lesbian, gay, bisexual, transgender, and queer or questioning health outcomes, significant health disparities continue to exist when compared with the heterosexual population.
- Sexual minorities tend to experience higher rates of numerous acute and chronic conditions than does the general population because of persistent stigma-associated stress.
- As a result of continued stigma and discrimination experienced in the health care setting, sexual minorities are significantly more likely to delay seeking medical care and are less likely to not have a consistent source for health care.
- A provider's failure to recognize and a person's lack of disclosure prevents vital discussions about human immunodeficiency virus risk, hormone therapy, cancer risk, hepatitis, and sexual health.
- Health care professionals have an ethical imperative to reduce discrimination and health care disparities for minority communities.

In recent decades, a great deal of attention has been placed on the reduction of health disparities that have plagued the lesbian, gay, bisexual, transgender, and queer or questioning (LGBTQ) community. Comprising more than 7% of the population in the United States, the National Institutes of Health identified the LGBTQ community as a heath disparity population and included sexual minority health in the Healthy People

The author declares no conflicts of interest.

This research did not receive any specific grant from funding agencies in the public, commercial, or not-for-profit sectors.

University of Wisconsin Oshkosh, College of Nursing, 800 Algoma Boulevard, Oshkosh, WI 54901, USA

E-mail address: englundh@uwosh.edu

2020 national initiative.[1] Similarly, reports from the US Department of Health and Human Services and the National Academy of Medicine (formerly the Institutes of Medicine) have underlined the unique health care needs of this growing population and called for policy changes and increase research in this area.[1] Despite growing attention being placed on LGBTQ health outcomes, significant health disparities continue to exist when compared with the heterosexual population.

There is a growing body of evidence illuminating the complex interactions between the multilevel minority stressors experienced by the LGBTQ community.[2–4] These interactions can limit employment opportunities, cause housing insecurities, and limit access to health care.[5] Only 21 states and the District of Columbia have antidiscrimination laws that specifically cover sexual orientation and gender identity.[6] This creates a situation where many LGBTQ individuals are working in states where they have no legal protection against discrimination in the workplace. Additionally, sexual minorities must navigate what is known as the lavender ceiling, which can be defined as an unofficial glass ceiling or upper limit of professional advancement for LGBTQ individuals.[7] Lavender ceilings are a social construct that result from pervasive bias and discrimination of sexual minorities in society.

Systemic biases, hostile work environments, and a lack of legal protection against discrimination may be contributing factors to why sexual minorities are twice as likely to be unemployed than are heterosexual individuals.[5] Undoubtedly, higher unemployment rates are a significant contributor to the fact that LGBTQ adults have higher poverty rates (21.6%) than do heterosexual individuals (15.7%), with the highest rates (29.4%) among transgender individuals.[8] Discrimination and stigma can contribute to housing insecurity for sexual minorities across a person's lifespan, from rejection by family and friends during one's youth to discrimination in the mortgage industry and rental market.[9] Higher poverty rates and discriminatory housing practices may help explain why less than half (49.8%) of LGBTQ adults own their homes compared with nearly 71% of non-LGBTQ adults.[9] Furthermore, sexual minorities are also disproportionately affected by homelessness across their lifespan, with up to 45% of all homeless adults identifying as a sexual minority.[9] LGBTQ youth and young adults are nearly 3 times more likely to be homeless than are their heterosexual counterparts.[8]

With regard to access to health care, passage of the Affordable Care Act (2010) significantly decreased the number of uninsured individuals in the United States. However, LGBTQ individuals continue to have higher uninsured rates (12.7%) when compared to the heterosexual population (11.4%) with comparable demographics.[10] Additionally, sexual minorities continue to experience numerous, less tangible barriers to health care that negatively impact health outcomes. For example, according to data obtained from the National Health Interview Survey, sexual minorities are significantly more likely to delay seeking medical care and are less likely to not have a consistent source for health care.[10]

## STIGMA AND DISCRIMINATION IN HEALTH CARE

Factors contributing to these findings include continued stigma and discrimination experienced in health care, as well as a lack of cultural competence and training regarding the unique health care needs of sexual minorities.[1,11,12] Stigma in the health care setting can range from overt discrimination, such as refusal of a health care provider to deliver care to a sexual minority patient, to inadvertent forms of bias including use of nonaffirming language and a lack of knowledge regarding LGBTQ health.[11,12] This knowledge gap may necessitate that sexual minorities take on the burdensome role of educator and inform providers about the unique health needs of the LGBTQ community. A lack of provider knowledge has also been shown to contribute to providers asking invasive and insensitive questions, and performing unnecessary or inappropriate laboratory tests, diagnostic tests, and examinations.[1,12]

Although attitudes regarding the LGBTQ population are slowly evolving to become less overtly tied to negative stereotypes, there remains a deeply rooted assumption of heteronormativity that continues to pervade society. Heteronormativity speaks to the assumption that heterosexuality is the norm or the only sexuality of individuals and society.[13] To compound the issue, many health care providers practice under this assumption and rarely ask clarifying questions regarding gender identity and sexual health.[13] This misassumption may lead sexual minorities to hide their sexual orientation and choose to not disclose their sexual status to health care providers.[11,13]

Failure to elicit a patient's gender identity and sexual orientation is analogous to a health care provider's failure to perform a health screening or diagnose a disease process.[1] In other words, eliciting a person's preferred gender and sexual orientation should be an integral component of any health visit. When providers assume heteronormativity with their patients, they are remiss in providing appropriate patient wellness and disease prevention strategies.[1] A provider's failure to recognize and a person's lack of disclosure prevents vital discussions about human immunodeficiency virus (HIV) risk, hormone therapy, cancer risk, hepatitis, and sexual health.[13,14]

## MINORITY STRESS IN THE LESBIAN, GAY, BISEXUAL, TRANSGENDER, AND QUEER OR QUESTIONING POPULATION

A review of the literature suggests that sexual minorities tend to experience higher rates of numerous acute and chronic conditions than the general population because of persistent stigma-associated stress.[2,3,14] The largest source of minority stress is structural stigma, which can be defined as the societal processes and structures in places that deny members of the LGBTQ community the same rights and opportunities provided for the heterosexual population.[3] Structural stigma facilitates discrimination in every aspect of a person's life including school, workplace, religious communities, and family. Both overt and covert forms of discrimination and stigmatization elevate the mental health burden experienced by members of the LGBTQ community, thus lowering the threshold for several acute and chronic conditions including substance abuse, risky sexual behaviors, and mental illness.[3]

LGBTQ-specific minority stressors can act synergistically across multiple levels to negatively impact the health status of an individual. For example, a Black bisexual man may experience stressors related to his status as both a racial and sexual minority. The additive stressors associated with poverty, housing insecurities, and poor access to health care further exacerbate health disparities.[3] Research suggests that the average lifespan of a LGBTQ individual who experiences unyielding structural stigma and minority stress can be prematurely decreased by more than a decade because of cardiovascular disease, depression, anxiety, tobacco use, alcohol and drug use, and suicidality. Furthermore, empiric evidence suggests that major depression is strongly associated with high disease burden as measured by the number of years a person lives with disability.[2,15]

## IMPACT OF MINORITY STRESS ON HEALTH OUTCOMES

When discussing health disparities associated with sexual orientation, it is important to consider the unique personal and social considerations that change as one ages. Specifically, there are certain risk factors that are more prevalent in a given life stage than in others. For example, research findings suggest that anxiety and depression peak in incidence and prevalence around 20 to 24 years of age.[4] Late adolescence and early adulthood tend to be the time that most LGBTQ individuals navigate coming out to their friends and family as a sexual minority. Disclosure of one's sexual identity can lead to feelings of intense stress and anxiety, and being subjected to rejection and loss of important personal relationships.[4] Moreover, LGBTQ individuals in late adolescence and early adulthood who disclose their sexual orientation may still be dealing with the deleterious effects of being exposed to aggression and bullying at school. Increased anxiety and depression in late adolescence and early adulthood may also be a contributing factor as to why alcohol and other drug use disorders are so prevalent during this time. Research suggests that alcohol use and other drug use peak during this time frame and then tend to dissipate as one ages.[4] This trajectory most likely mimics the relationship between drug use and mental health disorders, as individuals with illnesses such as anxiety and depression are 2 to 3 times more likely to abuse alcohol and drugs than those individuals who do not have mental health disorders.[4]

Empiric evidence suggests that youth and young adult sexual minorities are disproportionately affected by HIV/acquired immunodeficiency syndrome (AIDS) when compared with other generations of LGBTQ individuals.[16] According to the US Centers for Disease Control and Prevention, individuals between the ages of 13 and 24 accounted for 20% (6,135) of new HIV diagnoses in the United States.[16] Unfortunately, significant risk disparities exist, with young gay and bisexual men comprising nearly 85% of all new HIV diagnoses in 2020.[16] Young gay and bisexual men who are affected by depression, anxiety, and substance use issues are at an even greater risk for HIV and other sexually transmitted infections.[3,15] For example, anxiety and depression can increase HIV risk behaviors through disengagement, unhealthy coping, and inadequate implementation of health prevention behaviors. Anxiety and depression are associated with poor condom use; specifically, gay and bisexual men with post-traumatic stress disorder (PTSD) are 3 times more likely to report recent condomless intercourse compared to those without PTSD.[3]

Young and young adult LGBTQ individuals also face greater exposure to violence and victimization. Gay and bisexual males, as well as transgender females, are statistically more likely than their heterosexual counterparts to experience intimate partner violence (IPV).[17] Research suggests that 1 in 3 men have experienced physical violence, sexual violence, and/or stalking by an intimate partner.[17] The psychological impact of IPV for these populations can be compounded by their sexuality through the use of outing, coercive use of HIV/AIDS status, and destructive gendered stereotypes.[17] These gendered stereotypes and biases act as a barrier to postviolence services, as men and transgender females who seek help from health care agencies, hotlines, and law enforcement are often exposed to ridicule, blame, disbelief, or cast as the abuser.[18] Furthermore, the physical and emotional injuries sustained by sexual minority males and transgender females tend to be ignored or minimized.[18] As a result, victims can often experience the effects of a double closet, in that they not only feel compelled to keep their sexual orientation a secret, but their victimization of abuse also.[17] Both a failure to disclose and a lack of validation of a person's experiences with IPV can lead to substance abuse, depression, suicidality, and PTSD.[17]

The deleterious effects of sustained exposure to minority stressors become increasingly apparent as LGBTQ individuals age. Research suggests that middle-aged (36–55 years of age) and older men (56 years or older) who are a sexual minority are at a significantly higher risk for cardiovascular disease (CVD) than are heterosexual men.[4] Disparities in cardiovascular health may be reflective of a person's life accumulation of minority stress and those behaviors associated with exposure to chronic stress such as alcohol, tobacco, and other drug use.[4] Research suggests that middle-aged and older adults tend to have higher rates of obesity, as well as alcohol, tobacco, and drug abuse when compared with heterosexual and younger LGBTQ individuals.[14] HIV status can also increase a person's risk for CVD because of cardiometabolic changes and dyslipidemia associated with certain HIV treatment.[2,19] Additionally, recent studies have shown that the use of gender-affirming hormone therapy used for transgender women can contribute to poor cardiovascular health.[2,19]

The experiences of older LGBTQ adults have largely been absent from medical and nursing scholarship. What evidence exists suggests that this population experiences disproportionately poorer health outcomes when compared with their heterosexual peers of the same age. Older LGBTQ individuals tend to internalize the homophobia, discrimination, and rejection schemas that they have been exposed to over the course of their lifetime, thus resulting in feelings of depression, anxiety, and low self-esteem/self-worth (Pachankis and colleagues, 2019).[3] Older LGBTQ adults may subsequently choose to avoid societal interactions or situations that exacerbate their minority stress. This aversion may help explain why older LGBTQ adults (especially men) tend to participate less in preventative health screenings and avoid seeking medical care for acute and chronic conditions when compared with heterosexual individuals.[20]

Older LGBTQ men have been disproportionately exposed to the HIV/AIDS epidemic in that more than half of the nearly 1.2 million individuals living with HIV in the United States are 50 years of age or older.[16,21] The male-to-female ratio of older individuals living with HIV/AIDS in the United States is approximately 4:1.[21] The lack of health care organizations' commitment to research and support gay men affected with HIV and AIDS in the 1980s and 1990s has led to feelings of mistrust by older HIV/AIDS-positive men in particular. During this time, the stigma associated with HIV/AIDS was pervasive and this population was dismissed as being irresponsible deviants who became infected after participating in inappropriate, unprotected casual inter-course.[22] As a result, the aging HIV/AIDS positive population may view the current health care system as ineffective, neglectful, and hostile.[22]

The older LGBTQ population is at greatest risk for economic insecurity, thus further hindering access to and utilization of the health care system.[20,22] The intersection of health disparities, coupled with financial insecurity, may necessitate that older LGBTQ adults rely more heavily on both formal and informal support systems. Empiric evidence suggests, however, that LGBTQ older adults tend to have a diminished sense of community belonging and fewer sources of social support than do heterosexual older adults.[14,20] Heterosexual older adults tend to utilize their families (eg, children, spouse, siblings) for care and support in their later years. LGBTQ older adults must often rely on nonfamilial individuals (eg, friends or paid caregivers) as they have a higher likelihood of estrangement from their biological families and are much less likely to have children.[14,20] Informal support systems may not be consistently available to LGBTQ older adults, which increases their risk for social isolation and depression.[14]

## RECOMMENDATIONS

Although many complex factors contribute to the health disparities that exist within the LGBTQ community, empiric evidence suggests that sexual minorities often avoid seeking health care because of the stigma, discrimination, and mistreatment experienced in the health care setting.[1,14,23] Members of the LGBTQ community consistently report a scarcity of health care providers with sufficient knowledge of LGBTQ health care needs as a significant barrier to quality health care.[12,23,24] This is not surprising, as medical and nursing schools across the United States spend an average of 2 to

5 hours total on LGBTQ-specific content.[11,24] Additionally, the heteronormative nature of the health care system has led to the widely held assumption that all individuals are heterosexual until they do or say something that negates this assumption. Heteronormative attitudes are deeply embedded within societal mores and may be hidden from conscious awareness.[12] Such a complex, multifaceted, and deeply rooted phenomenon requires health care leaders to utilize more innovative, sustained, and robust pedagogical approaches to education of medical and nursing students.

In an effort to address the pervasive health disparities experienced by the LGBTQ community, institutions of higher education have focused on implementing cultural competence curricula within their medical and nursing programs. Despite this attention, barriers continue to exist regarding the addition of more sustained and robust LGBTQ content in medical and nursing education. These barriers include a lack of trained faculty competent to teach LGBTQ topics, faculty perceptions that sexual minority health topics are not relevant to their specific courses, and limited instruction time.[1] Current programs aimed at improving cultural competence of medical and nursing students tend to be broadly defined and provide a more general approach to interacting with minoritized populations. The prevailing method of medical and nursing education tends to focus on mastering a number of discrete knowledge points regarding sexual minority health. Such a structure makes it difficult for students and faculty to assimilate and integrate this knowledge in a way that promotes understanding and cultural competence.[12,24]

With the expansion of LGBTQ-focused research, medical and nursing educators must implement specific didactic and clinical competencies across the curriculum rather than at discrete points.[1,25] Research has shown that medical and nursing students who are exposed to LGBTQ content early and consistently throughout the curriculum demonstrate greater proficiency in addressing the unique health care needs of LGBTQ patients.[23,25] Whether through simulation or live patient contact experiences, repeated exposure has been shown to result in significantly higher scores on knowledge, student satisfaction, self-confidence, and clinical performance measures when compared with single-exposure modalities.[11,23]

Educators must be systematic in their approach to inclusion of LGBTQ content in medical and nursing programs. The first step is to critically evaluate current curriculum and identify gaps in knowledge acquisition. Educators must then use a multimodal approach that goes beyond simply highlighting the health disparities that exist with regard to LGBTQ health outcomes. Educators must implement situated learning activities that are grounded in the concepts of equity, inclusion, and social justice.[25] It is also imperative that LGBTQ curriculum be structured within the paradigm of minority stress, and that learning activities focus on the complex and evolving interplay of structural stigma on health outcomes of sexual minorities. There are several problem-based learning activities and e-learning technologies readily available online (eg, lavenderhealth.org; glma.org) for educators to use. Guest speakers, such as members of the LGBTQ community, and health care professionals with expertise in sexual minority health have proven to be an effective means by which to discuss communication strategies, cultural competence, and heteronormativity.[11,25]

It is vital that nursing programs provide educators with opportunities to develop competence and confidence in teaching LGBTQ content. There is an expectation that all providers engage in activities that continually update their clinical knowledge on a wide range of health care topics. Enhancing one's skillset and behavioral domains of practice is typically accomplished through accredited continuing education training and programs. There are numerous LGBTQ continuing education opportunities available to medical and nursing professionals as a means to enhancing cultural competence. Unfortunately, there remains a barrier to LGBTQ continuing education trainings either reaching or being used by health care providers. Results of a national survey suggests that less than 20% of physician and nursing professionals reported participating in comprehensive training on LGBTQ health.[1] This suggests a lack of awareness of existing health disparities that affect sexual minorities, and/or limited self-awareness about biases and assumptions held by health care professionals towards LGBTQ individuals.[1] Health care organizations and universities must make LGBTQ health a priority and require a commitment to cultural competence through sustained continuing education and professional development.

## SUMMARY

Members of the LGBTQ community continue to experience homophobia, assumptions of heteronormativity, poor access to health care, and unequal or unsatisfactory health care treatment. Health care professionals have an ethical imperative to reduce discrimination and health care disparities for minority communities. Position statements put forth from several agencies including the American Association of Medical Colleges and the American Association of Colleges of Nursing have shed light on the gaps that continue to exist in physician and nursing education regarding LGBTQ health.[1] Similarly, both the Joint Commission and National Academy of Medicine call for the consistent inclusion of gender identity and sexual orientation information so as to facilitate a better understanding of the cultural needs of patients. Health care providers have a duty to be culturally competent, and to provide a safe and supportive environment within which patients can disclose crucial aspects of their health and social histories.

## CLINICS CARE POINTS

- Given the high incidence of HIV in some LGBTQ populations, HIV prevention constitutes a critical aspect of care for this population.
- It is imperative that providers recognize his/her own assumptions regarding gender identity and sexual orientation, and how these assumptions may impact the patient-provider dyad.
- Health care providers must consistently conduct depression/mental health screening and to be aware of resources for LGBTQ individuals in the local community.

## REFERENCES

1. Bonvicini KA. LGBTQ healthcare disparities: what progress have we made? Patient Educ Couns 2017;100:2357–61.
2. Caceres BA, Streed CG, Corliss HL, et al. Assessing and addressing cardiovascular health in LGBTQ adults. Circulation 2020;142:e321–32.
3. Pachankis JE, McConocha EM, Reynolds JS, et al. Project ESTEEM protocol: a randomized controlled trial oof an LGBTQ-affirmative treatment for young adult sexual minority men's mental and sexual health. BMC Public Health 2019;19:1–12.
4. Rice CE, Vasilenko SA, Fish JN, et al. Sexual minority health disparities: an examination of age-related trends across adulthood in a national cross-sectional sample. Ann Epidemiol 2019;31:20–5.
5. Charleton BM, Gordon AR, Reisner S, et al. Sexual orientation-related disparities in employment, health insurance, healthcare access and health-related quality of

life: a cohort study of US male and female adolescents and young adults. BJM Open 2018;8(5):e020418.

6. Brennan M., Livingston A., Gaitan V., Five facts about housing access for LGBT people 2018. Available at: https://housingmatters.urban.org/articles/five-facts-about-housing-access-lgbt-people. Accessed November 18, 2022.

7. Badgett MV, Carpenter CS, Sansone D. LGBTQ economics. J Econ Perspect 2021;35(2):141–70.

8. Badgett M.L., Choi S.K., & Wilson B.M., LGBT poverty in the United States: a study of differences between sexual orientation and gender identity groups. 2019. Available at: https://williamsinstitute.law.ucla.edu/wp-content/uploads/National-LGBT-Poverty-Oct-2019.pdf?utm_campaign=hsric&utm_medium=email&utm_source=govdelivery. Accessed November 18, 2022.

9. Romero A.P., Goldberg S.K. and Vasquez L.A., LGBT people and housing afford-ability, discrimination, and homelessness, 2020, The Williams Institute, UCLA, Los Angeles, CA, Available at: https://williamsinstitute.law.ucla.edu/wp-content/uploads/LGBT-Housing-Apr-2020.pdf. Accessed November 18, 2022.

10. Bosworth A., Turrini G., Pyda S., et al., Health insurance coverage and access to care for LGBTQ+ individuals: current trends and key challenges issue brief 2021. Available at: https://aspe.hhs.gov/sites/default/files/2021-07/lgbt-health-ib.pdf. Accessed November 18, 2022.

11. Englund H, Basler J, Meine K. Nursing education and inclusion of LGBTQ topics: making strides or falling short? Nurse Educat 2020;45(4):182–4.

12. Hsieh N, Shuster SM. Health and health care of sexual and gender minorities. J Health Soc Behav 2021;62(3):318–33.

13. Stewart K, O'Reilly P. Exploring the attitudes, knowledge and beliefs of nurses and midwives of the healthcare needs of the LGBTQ population: an integrative review. Nurse Educ Today 2017;53:67–77.

14. Medina-Martinez J, Saus-Ortega C, Sanchez-Lorente MM, et al. Health inequities in LGBTQ people and nursing interventions to reduce them: a systematic review. IJERPH 2021;18(22):1–16.

15. Paley A., The Trevor Project: national survey on LGBTQ youth mental health. 2021. Available at: https://www.thetrevorproject.org/wp-content/uploads/2021/05/The-Trevor-Project-National-Survey-Results-2021.pdf. Accessed November 18, 2022.

16. Centers for Disease Control and Prevention. Diagnoses of HIV infection in the United States and dependent areas, 2020. HIV Surveillance Report 2020. Available at: https://www.cdc.gov/hiv/library/reports/hiv-surveillance/vol-33/index.html. Accessed November 18, 2022.

17. Dickerson-Amaya N, Coston BM. Invisibility is not invincibility: the impact of inti-mate partner violence on gay, bisexual, and straight men's mental health. Amer-ican J Mens Health 2019;13(3):1–12.

18. Donne MD, DeLuca J, Pleskach P, et al. Barriers to and facilitators of help-seeking among men who experience sexual violence. AM Mens Health 2018; 12(2):189–201.

19. Connelly PJ, Freel EM, Perry C, et al. Gender-affirming hormone therapy, vascular health and cardiovascular disease in transgender adults. Hypertension 2019;74: 1266–74.

20. Putney JM, Keary S, Hebert N, et al. Fear runs deep: the anticipated needs of LGBT older adults in long-term care. J Gerontol Soc Work 2018;61(8):887–907.

21. Autenreith CS, Beck EJ, Stelzle D, et al. Global and regional trends of people living with HIV aged 50 and over: estimates and projections for 2000-2020. PLoS One 2018;1–11. https://doi.org/10.1371/journal.pone.0207005.
22. Kia H. Subjugation and resistance in older gay men's health care experiences. Toronto, CA: University of Toronto; 2019. Doctoral dissertation.
23. Parke JA, Safer JD. Clinical exposure to transgender medicine improves students' preparedness above levels seen with didactic teaching alone: a key addition to the Boston University Model for teaching transgender Healthcare. Transgender Health 2018;3(1):10–6.
24. Korpaisarn S, Safer JD. Gaps in transgender medical education among healthcare providers: a major barrier to care for transgender persons. Rev Endocr Metab Disord 2018;19:1–5.
25. McCann E, Brown M. The inclusion of LGBT+ health issues within undergraduate healthcare education and professional training programmes: a systematic review. Nurse Educ Today 2018;64:204–14.

# Male Caregiving
## It Often Looks Different

Jason Mott, PhD, RN

### KEYWORDS

- Caregiving • Male caregiving • Nursing history

### KEY POINTS

- Men view the care provider role as a job and will treat it that way.
- Men want to be competent in the tasks that they need to complete and view their masculinity on their competency.
- Men need to be provided education related to the caregiving role so that they can function at the highest level possible.
- Health care providers need to understand the differences that men bring to the caregiving role and try to understand where they are coming from.

Nursing is a profession of providing care. Henderson[1] stated that nurses help individuals sick or well in the performance of those activities contributing to health, its recovery (or to a peaceful death) that those persons would do for themselves if they had the requisite strength, will or knowledge, and to do so as to help them become independent of such help as rapidly as possible. When one thinks about caregiving, many images may come to mind. It could be the mother sitting with their sick child. It could be the nurse sitting at the patient's bedside holding their hand as they are dying. The one commonality that exists is that this individual is typically female. The image of caring and providing care usually does not contain the male nurse being competent in their care. Even though they have been providing care for thousands of years, males are often not pictured when describing caregiving. This article will examine the history of male caregiving, traits of male caregivers, and practical approaches that can be used to support male caregivers.

### HISTORY

Providing care to others has existed since the dawn of time. Traditionally, women have been socialized in the caregiving role. Girls took babysitting classes, whereas boys were coached by their fathers in outdoor activities and athletics. Often, boys are taught to be dominant and not to show emotional vulnerability, whereas girls are

College of Nursing, University of Wisconsin Oshkosh, 800 Algoma Boulevard, Oshkosh WI 54901, USA
E-mail address: mottj@uwosh.edu

Nurs Clin N Am 58 (2023) 505–512
https://doi.org/10.1016/j.cnur.2023.06.009
0029-6465/23/© 2023 Elsevier Inc. All rights reserved.

taught to be sensitive to the needs of others, which is often viewed as caring behavior.[2] Therefore, males have not been viewed traditionally as being caregivers. However, that is changing.

According to AARP,[3] more than 50 million provided unpaid care to a family member in the United States. Accius[4] found that approximately 40% of family caregivers are male, which equates to roughly 16 million males. In the nursing profession, about 14% of the 3 million nurses are male, which equates to approximately 426,000.[5] These numbers show that the numbers of male caregivers are increasing.

In order to truly understand the roots of nursing, we must first look at the history of men in nursing. Nursing care has been around for centuries. As previously stated, men typically provided nursing care to outsiders. The first known people trained in nursing were men during the Hippocratic period of ancient Greece. These men served as assistants to the physician, while women often cared for those within the home. This was due the role of society which banned women to the home.[6] The first recorded school of nursing was established in 250 B.C. in India.[7] In this school, only men were considered pure enough to become nurses. Requirements of these male nurses included:

*Of good behavior, distinguished for purity, possessed of cleverness and skill, imbued with kindness, skilled in every service a patient may require, competent to cook food, skilled in bathing and washing the patient, rubbing and massaging the limbs, lifting and assisting him to walk about, well skilled in making and cleansing of beds, readying the patient and skillful in waiting upon one that is ailing and never unwilling to do anything that may be ordered*[7]

In ancient Rome, military hospitals were built to provide the best medical care to soldiers. During this time, a group of male nurses called the nosocomi, were employed to care for wounded and sick soldiers.[6] These men continued providing medical care for Roman soldiers until the fall of the Roman Empire.

The tradition of men as nurses continued throughout the first several centuries A.D. Most of the time, men acting in the role of nurses were associated with military or religious orders. These men provided nursing care during military conflicts as well as during the many plagues that swept across Europe during the Middle Ages. There are several different groups that have been associated with nursing during these time periods.

Early religious orders of nurses included the Benedictines and Alexians. These groups would start hospitals to care for sick individuals. However, it was during the Byzantine era that nursing care started to move from care being provided by monks to having paid nurses provide nursing care. Again, men were primarily in the role of the nurse, except due to societal regulations, women provided intimate care for female patients.[6]

The Alexian Brothers were formed in the 14th century to care for individuals during the black plague in Germany. They would provide care for the sick, feed the hungry, and bury the dead. Because of widespread fear of the plague, these individuals were forced outside the city gates. The Alexian Brothers would leave the city to care for these individuals. They were often viewed as heretics during their early history, as their approach was unconventional for the time period. They first became an official religious order in 1472. The group practiced in Europe for several more centuries. They also began a ministry in the United States in 1866, where they began to care for victims of a cholera epidemic in Chicago. They were noted for their compassion and professional expertise. The health care ministry they founded in Chicago continues to this day, as well as ministries in Belgium, England, Ireland, and Germany.[8]

There are 2 religious men who are heavily associated with the nursing profession during the Middle Ages. These 2 saints, St. John of God and St. Camillus de Lellis, were both soldiers who became to nurses. Juan de Mena was a friar who is associated with nursing in North America.

St. John of God is the patron saint of booksellers, printers, heart patients, hospitals, nurses, the sick, and firefighters. An impulsive man born in the early 1500s, John, followed many different paths before becoming a nurse. He followed a priest from an early age. He also worked as a shepherd and was a soldier in 2 separate wars. During this time, he worked for a wealthy family and nursed them back to health when they fell ill. At one point in his life, he was committed to a mental health facility, where he was tied down and beaten every day for 40 days. After being moved within the hospital, he nursed sick patients to health. At that time, he also decided to found his own hospital, begging for money and supplies.[9] He was known to care for the mentally ill, homeless, crippled, and abandoned children.[7]

St. Camillus de Lillus is the other saint of the sick and nurses. Once a soldier, he had many problems with gambling that forced him to reexamine his life. After his unit disbanded, and suffering from an incurable leg wound he received during his time as a solider, he was placed in a hospital for incurable individuals. During this time, de Lillus began to care for other patients in the hospital. Seeing the poor care they received, he decided to build his own hospital. De Lillus, along with other holy men, would care for the sick. They could be seen wearing a red cross on their back. This symbol is still used as the symbol of the International Red Cross. He was passionate about caring for others and insisted on the cleanliness and technical competence of the caregivers working for him. He is also credited with creating the first military field ambulance.[10]

Friar Juan de Mena is the first nurse in the United States. He arrived in the United States, on the gulf coast of Texas, 70 years before the pilgrims arrived. He cared for the sick in Mexico for years before being called back to Spain, where he later died.[11]

### American Civil War

During the American Civil War, there were many famous individuals who served as "nurses." The interesting part related to men in nursing during the Civil War was that they were not allowed to be called nurses, even though they were the individuals providing much of the care to wounded soldiers. This was due to much of the training that was received. Before the American Civil war, men were enlisted as and functioned in the role of assistive medical personnel.[12] This was congruent with how nursing had been practiced up until this point, where men were trained by surgeons.[13]

The confederate army assigned 30 men per regiment to nurse and care for the wounded soldiers as well as removed those who could not walk from the battlefield.[14] Famous poet Walt Whitman served as a nurse and wrote 2 poems from the view of the male nurse during the civil war.[14] Like previously stated, men caring for the sick and injured during the civil war were not allowed to be called nurses. That title was only for women who were organized by Dorothea Dix.[14]

Dix served during the Civil War as the Union army's Superintendent of Female Nurses. It was in this role that Dix recruited women into the role of nurse. At the time, she was put in charge of all female nurses in the Union Army. By the end of the Civil War, she had recruited 3000 women to serve as Union Nurses.[15]

The first time that a woman was mentioned as a nurse in the United States was in 1890.[7] In 1896, a delegate of 20 female nurses gather in New York City to form the Nurses Associated Alumnae of the United States and Canada.[16] This group, which became the American Nurses Association (ANA) in 1911,[16] excluded men from joining its ranks.[17] It was not until 1930 that bylaws were amended to allow men to become members of the ANA.[18] Men did not join the ANA until 1940.[12]

Men were excluded from attending nursing schools, except for the few nursing schools for men. This primarily occurred in stated funded schools.[19] This exclusion of men from nursing schools continued in many institutions until the early 1980s.[19] In fact, in 1960, 85% of nursing schools excluded the admittance of men into their program based solely on their gender.[17] Next, characteristics of male caregivers will be explored.

## MALE CAREGIVERS

Male caregivers have been found to have a specific set of traits that differ from their female counterparts. The most common trait of male caregivers found in the literature was that they bring a unique set of masculine behaviors to the care they provide. Male caregivers demonstrate caring by highlighting the practical tasks they perform, the technical skills they possess, and their ability to take control of the situation.[20] Male caregivers will tend to take on a problem-centered approach to caregiving and see the role as challenges to overcome. They will view their role as being a protector or provider.[20] Males in the caregiving role tend to be autonomous, meaning that they prefer to have independence over situations. In fact, being autonomous and demonstrating independence in the caregiving role allows the male to demonstrate competence as both as man and a caregiver.[20]

Although they often prefer to be autonomous, that doesn't mean that male caregivers don't want support or education. Mott and colleagues[20] found a variety of responses from male caregivers in response to social support. In general, research findings related to the acceptance of support by male caregivers are mixed and require further study. Some authors found that men refuse all types of support, especially formal community support. Other men were willing to accept support, but that support came more in the form of unpaid family or friend support. Yet, in other studies, men were very willing to receive any type of support.[20]

Men did not always receive support when they asked for it, thus making it less likely for them to seek support in the future. Men who sought assistance may be perceived as weak, or as lacking need of assistance. What men find useful is information about how to provide care, skill development, and how to perform the role of caregiver. Oftentimes, men felt bewildered and didn't know where to begin when taking on the role of caregiver.[20]

There are limited outlets for male family caregivers. As a result, they are at a greater risk of social isolation. In many cases, male family caregivers are no longer able or willing to socialize with their friends due to caregiving commitment, or feel like they need to withdraw in order to focus all their energy on the person for which they were caring. When men received social support, their caregiver role strain/stress was diminished, and they were less likely to be isolated.[20]

Many male caregivers want and need education. AARP[4] reported that 72% of male family caregivers do not really know how to provide care, and 58% of male family caregivers would like a qualified person to show them how to perform the tasks they need to do. In addition, about half of men (49%) prefer hands-on training with a qualified person observing them.[4] Mott and colleagues[20] discovered that male caregivers are interested in "do-it-yourself home kits, networking opportunities, community-specific information regarding resources, and in-home assessments of needs. Also, men need disease-specific education. For instance, "when caring for a loved one with Alzheimer disease, men need specific information related to the disease and what to look for as the disease progresses."[20(pE22)].

The need for education is so great that the Caregiver Advise, Record, Enable Act (CARE) was passed by 39 states and mandates that hospitals or rehabilitation facilities explain and provide demonstrations of medical tasks to family caregivers.[21] The RAISE Family Caregivers Act requires the secretary of Health and Human Services to develop, maintain, and update a strategy to recognize and support caregivers.[22]

The final trait of male caregivers focuses on the emotional aspects of caregiving. When discussing male family caregivers, this focuses on caregiver role strain. Most research found that women experience or report higher incidence of role strain. It is theorized that men report less caregiver role strain due to their approach to caregiving. Several authors discovered that taking a problem-focused approach to caregiving, such as men do, decreases perceived role strain.[20] Others postulated that men experience the same amount of caregiver role strain as females, but report it less often to appear masculine and that they can "handle anything."[20] Finally, practical approaches that male caregivers can use will be addressed.

## PRACTICAL APPROACHES

There are many practical approaches that can be provided to male caregivers (**Table 1**). These are based on many of the things that male caregivers want and need from their providers and support people. The largest need for male caregivers is education.

When providing education, there are several important aspects to include. Provide as much information about the disease as possible. This may include what to expect during the course of disease progression, challenges that may arise, and how to overcome those challenges. Male caregivers should be provided with hands-on demonstrations for any of the skills that they may need to provide. They should be encouraged to ask questions and seek out clarification as needed. One additional method of education that has been shown to be beneficial is to find other males who are going through similar circumstances and bounce ideas off of one another.

| Table 1 Characteristics and practical implications | |
| --- | --- |
| **Characteristic** | **Practical Implication** |
| Masculinization of care | 1. Understand where the man is coming from<br>2. Understand how men typically approach the caregiving role<br>3. Ask what their needs are<br>4. Provide education<br>  a. Medications<br>  b. What to discuss at appointments<br>  c. What to expect with disease progression<br>  d. How to perform the tasks they need to<br>  e. Support services available<br>  f. How to be an advocate for themselves and the person they are caring for |
| Social support | 1. Ask the man what their support needs are.<br>2. Be willing to offer whatever support they feel they need.<br>3. Encourage them to meet with other men in similar circumstances.<br>4. Provide community resources<br>5. Try to limit social isolation |
| Caregiver role strain | 1. Allow the male caregivers time to talk about what they are experiencing.<br>2. Provide resources for them.<br>3. Understand that they might not be experiencing role strain.<br>4. Financial support may be necessary, as many caregivers will decrease the amount of time they are working to provide caregiving services. |

It is also important for male caregivers to be comfortable with asking for help and taking a break. Oftentimes, these caregivers may feel like they are being held hostage in the situation. They don't want to relinquish control over the care they are providing and become stuck in that role. They need to be allowed to take a break, to know that it is ok. They should also be encouraged to use available resources.

One area that is often a struggle for male caregivers is navigating the health care system. Too often, men allow their significant others to navigate health care for them, or don't take ownership in their own health care. Then, when they are tasked with navigating the health care system for someone else, they have a difficult time doing so. Male caregivers should be provided with information as to how to navigate the health care system. They should be informed to come prepared for appointments.

Appointment preparation includes many different things. They should know what medications that are prescribed and if they are being taken appropriately. If there are struggles with the patient's ability or willingness to take medications, those should be discussed as well. The male caregiver should be instructed to write down any changes that they are seeing with the person they are providing care for. They should also write down any questions that they may have as they arise, so they don't get flustered or forget to ask the questions that they had.

When talking with the provider, the male caregiver should not be afraid to speak up. They should provide information about what they need from the provider or interaction. They should help the provider understand where they are coming from. They should also explain to the provider their view of the caregiving role. This will allow the caregiver and provider to be on the same page in terms of wants, needs, and expectations.

Within the health care system, the male caregiver should be encouraged to be an advocate. This means they should not only advocate for the person that they are providing care for, but should also advocate for themselves, whether that is asking for additional education or just letting the providers know what they need. If they are struggle in the role, they should be partnered with a social worker, who can provide many resources for them to take advantage of. They need to know that they are not in it alone.

When the care recipient is in the health care environment, it is important for the caregiver to provide as much information about that individual as possible. The health care team should be provided information about the client, what works and doesn't work for them, and what their primary needs are. The caregiver should also provide information about themselves, like how they provide care, what their needs are and what their expectations are.

Peer support has been shown to be a vital component of providing support for male family caregivers.[23] Although group sessions do not tend to work, what is effective are activities done with other men experiencing similar paths. This might include playing golf or having dinner with other caregivers. It's typically men doing male activities together in order to relieve stress and have an emotional outlet. It is also critical to teach men that reaching out for help is not a sign of weakness. Although most male caregivers agree that caregiving is stressful, very few seek help; they often avoid talking about their situation with others don't feel comfortable discussing the emotional challenges of caregiving and they then struggle in the role due to a lack of support. Groups such as Jack's Caregiver Coalition can help men connect with other men going through a similar situation.

## SUMMARY

As men take on more of a caregiving role in society, the need to understand how they provide care continues to grow. It is imperative that nurses understand the needs of men in the caregiving role as well as how they provide care differently than their female counterparts. Education related to caregiving needs to be individualized to best meet the needs of those providing and receiving care.

Also, more research needs to be done related to men in the caregiving role. The research related to men in the caregiving role is limited. It is critical to understand the needs of male caregivers. It is also important to understand the challenges and barriers that they face on a daily basis in providing care. If male caregivers can be better supported, it will only help to improve the health of the community in general.

## CLINICS CARE POINTS

- Educate men on the importance of advocacy.
- Help men understand what they need to do in a situation.
- Demonstrate care activities to the male caregiver.

## DISCLOSURE

The author has nothing to disclose.

## REFERENCES

1. Henderson V. The nature of nursing: a definition and its implications, practice, research, and education. Macmillan Company; 1966.
2. Cancian FM, Oliker SJ. Caring and gender. Pine Forge Press; 2000.
3. AARP. Caregiving in the United States 2020. Published May 14, 2020. Available at: https://www.aarp.org/ppi/info-2020/caregiving-in-the-united-states.html. Accessed February 2, 2023.
4. Accius J. Breaking Stereotypes: Spotlight on Male Family Caregivers. AARP Public Policy Institute. Published March 2017. Available at: https://www.aarp.org/content/dam/aarp/ppi/2017-01/Breaking-Stereotypes-Spotlight-on-Male-Family-Caregivers.pdf. Accessed February 2, 2023.
5. Nurse Demographics and Statistics in the United States. Zippia.com. Updated September 9, 2022. Available at: https://www.zippia.com/nurse-jobs/demographics/. Accessed February 2, 2023.
6. O'Lynn CE, Tranbarger RE. Men in nursing: history, challenges, and opportunities. Springer; 2007.
7. Howard G. What do you know about the history of nursing? Ala Nurse 2008; 35(2):4.
8. Alexian Brothers. Congregation of Alexian Brothers History. Published 2017. Available at: http://www.alexianbrothers.org/aboutus/congregation-of-alexian-brothers-history/. Accessed February 2, 2023.
9. Catholic Online. St. John of God. Published 2022. Available at: https://www.catholic.org/saints/saint.php?saint_id=68. Accessed February 2, 2023.
10. Franciscan Media. Saint Camillus de Lellis. Published 2023. Available at: https://www.franciscanmedia.org/saint-of-the-day/saint-camillus-de-lellis/. Accessed February 2, 2023.
11. Menstuff. Men and Nursing. Published 2023. Available at: http://www.menstuff.org/issues/byissue/malenurses.html. Accessed February 2, 2023.

12. Carleton E. Nurse Corps Fought to Include Male Nurses as Officers. U.S. Army. Published January 31, 2019. Available at: https://www.army.mil/article/216814/nurse_corps_fought_to_include_male_nurses_as_officers. Accessed February 2, 2023.

13. Brown B, Nolan PW, Crawford P. Men in Nursing: Ambivalence in Care, Gender and Masculinity. Available at: http://www.brown.uk.com/publications/MEN.htm. Accessed February 2, 2023.

14. Ford M. A brined history of Men in Nursing. Published 2019. Available at: https://www.nursingtimes.net/news/research-and-innovation/focus-a-brief-history-of-men-in-nursing-06-03-2019/. Accessed February 2, 2023.

15. Dorothea Dix 1802-1887. Civilwarhome.com. Published 2014. Available at: http://www.civilwarhome.com/dixbio.html. Accessed February 2, 2023.

16. American Nurses Association. The History of the American Nurses Association. Available at: https://www.nursingworld.org/ana/about-ana/history/. Accessed February 2, 2023.

17. Rischer K. Men in Nursing. KeithRN. Published February 13, 2019. Available at: https://www.keithrn.com/2019/02/men-in-nursing/. Accessed February 2, 2023.

18. American Nurses Association. Historical Review. Nursing World. Available at: https://www.nursingworld.org/~48de6f/globalassets/docs/ana/ana-expandedhistoricalreview.pdf. Accessed February 2, 2023.

19. Chung V. Men in Nursing. Allnurses.com. Published February 25, 2005. Available at: https://allnurses.com/men-nursing-article-t69840. Accessed February 2, 2023.

20. Mott J, Schmidt B, MacWilliams B. Male caregivers: shifting roles among family caregivers. Clin J Oncol Nurs 2019;23(1):E17–24.

21. AARP 2014 State Law to Help Family Caregivers. Available at: https://www.aarp.org/politics-society/advocacy/caregiving-advocacy/info-2014/aarp-creates-model-state-bill.html. Accessed February 2, 2023.

22. AARP. RAISE Act Promises Federal Help for Family Caregivers. Updated September 30, 2021. Available at: https://www.aarp.org/politics-society/advocacy/caregiving-advocacy/info-2015/raise-family-caregivers-act.html. Accessed February 2, 2023.

23. AARP. The hidden male caregiver. Updated 2017. Available at: https://www.aarp.org/caregiving/life-balance/info-2017/hidden-male-caregiver.html. Accessed February 2, 2023.

# Risk Factors for Suicide in Men

Vernon M. Langford, DNP, APRN, FNP-C*

## KEYWORDS

- Risk factors • Suicide attempt • Suicide • Suicidal behavior • Male • Men

## KEY POINTS

- Suicide is among the leading causes of death in the United States and globally.
- Men have an increased mortality rate from suicide compared with women.
- Awareness, clinical screening, and interventions targeted at risk factors impacting suicidal behavior in men could aid clinicians in reducing their incidence of suicide.
- The complex pathophysiology of suicidality in men includes many contributing factors, but health care professionals may assist in helping recognize and manage many of these.
- There are available screening tools and interventions that have shown reliability in detecting and reducing the ideation and completion of suicide.

## INTRODUCTION

A leading cause of preventable death and disability in both the United States and worldwide, suicide is a critical problem that cannot be ignored in either the public health landscape or the societal discourse.[1–6] Suicide is defined as death caused by injurious behavior that was directed at oneself with the intent to die as a result.[2–4] This is different from a suicide attempt, which is nonfatal and can range in severity, but is also self-directed with the intention of dying via behavior that is potentially injurious, although no injury may actually be sustained in the process.[3,6] The term suicidal behavior or suicidality is more encompassing and can include both an attempt and the suicide itself.[7] Suicidal ideations, however, may be referred to as suicidal ideas or suicidal thoughts, and include more broadly a variety of thoughts, desires, and obsessions with death and suicide.[,8] Increased incidence of suicidal ideations and suicidal behaviors are often linked to psychiatric/mental health disorders but not exclusively.[8,9]

Suicide literacy relates to possessing the understanding of the causes, recognizable signs, and available treatments involved with suicide risk.[10] Suicide signs or warning signs are indications of current suicidal behavior either witnessed or reported, and

Citrus State Healthcare Consultants, PLLC
* 1070 Montgomery, Suite 2306, Altamonte Springs, FL 32714
*E-mail address:* Vernon.Langford@hotmail.com

Nurs Clin N Am 58 (2023) 513–524
https://doi.org/10.1016/j.cnur.2023.06.010
0029-6465/23/© 2023 Elsevier Inc. All rights reserved.

they point to a potential risk of suicide within a specified period of time in the near future.[10,11] There are numerous risk factors and triggering variables connected to adult suicide in the general population, and risk factors for suicide can change throughout one's life.[8] Despite much research being conducted with regard to suicidality and risk factors in general, by comparison to age, socioeconomic status, ethnicity or geographic location, little research has targeted the risk factors of gender-specific suicidality related to men. As such, attempting to predict with significant certainty who will act on suicidal plans and who may simply briefly consider the ideation of suicide is difficult.[1,2,5,12]

## EPIDEMIOLOGY

Worldwide, the World Health Organization (WHO) reported that in 2019, suicide was responsible for the death of approximately 703,000 people each year, with an age-standardized suicide rate of 9.0 suicides per 100,000 persons in 2019 (average of <2–80 suicides per 100,000 persons).[13,14] Comparing males to females globally, the age-standardized suicide rate was markedly 2.3 times higher for males (12.6 suicides versus 5.4 per 100 000 persons).[14] Despite variance in income for countries, men sustained higher suicide rates compared to women worldwide, with suicide as the fourth leading cause of death for those aged 15 to 29 years.[14] The US Centers for Disease Control and Prevention (CDC) list suicide as the eleventh leading cause of death, with a rate of 14.5 suicides per 100,000 persons in 2021.[15] Looking historically at CDC data, the suicide rate steadily increased from 2000 to 2018, declined from 2018 to 2020 (14.2 suicides per 100,000 persons versus 13.5 suicides per 100,000 persons) before increasing once more in 2021 (14.5 suicides per 100,000 persons,) with the most common method of suicide being firearm-related for both women and men in 2020 (1.8 suicides per 100,000 persons versus 12.5 suicides per 100,000 persons).[16–18]

One reason for such a noticeable difference in rates when comparing males to females is due to men completing suicides more often despite women attempting suicide more often. This is referred to as the gender paradox and is related to a myriad of factors such as methods used when attempting suicide (firearms for men versus poisoning and suffocation for women) as well as childhood experiences, coping mechanisms, social/biological/cultural factors, and emotional feelings/behavior.[2,19] Contrasting suicide attempts and completed suicides, suicide attempts can occur up to 30 times more often than completions, while completions are 3 times more likely in men, although these numbers are likely much worse if accounting for under-reporting.[20] There is no known country where men do not outnumber women for completed suicide.[2]

## RISK FACTORS

With clinicians trained to provide patient-centered care, presentation of suicidality in the male population not being well studied inhibits the incorporation of male-specific screening guidelines and treatments as a standardized clinical practice guideline.[10,21,22] There are many clinical practice guidelines in use today from reputable clinical organizations, but none address both who is most at risk and when they are most likely to by acutely influenced toward suicide when capturing risk factor and warning sign data for men.[10,11,21,22] A systematic review by Richardson, Robb, and O'Connor from 2021 found 68 risk factors in the prospective and retrospective studies selected and subdivided them into the groups of sociodemographic factors (19), mental health/psychiatric illness (16), characteristics of suicidal behavior (3), physical health/illness (13), negative life events/trauma (11), and psychological factors (6).[2] These factors were compiled into **Tables 1** and **2** as they comprise the most comprehensive list to date.

Not surprisingly, many of the same risk factors exist for adults in general and with variances in gender effect when assessing available psychological autopsy literature.[23–26] There may be other risk factors that tend to have disproportional impacts on men, but often a there is a lack of analysis stratification to demonstrate such a relationship in the data.[23] One such separate element to consider is the adherence to masculine norms such as high self-reliance, which can create additional psychological stress and be a risk factor for suicidal ideation.[27] Another factor would be the release from incarceration, which increases the risk for men and women.[28] If focusing more broadly on the subgroups of risk factors provided by the aforementioned systematic review, a clearer picture of where and how to target risk factors for suicide emerges.

**Table 1**
**Personal factors contributing to increased suicide risk in men**

| Risk Subgroup | Risk Factors | |
|---|---|---|
| Sociodemographic characteristics | 1. Being divorced, widowed, separated, or single<br>2. Same sex married relationship<br>3. Being unemployed<br>4. Low household income as a child<br>5. Social and material deprivation<br>6. Living alone<br>7. Small circle of friends<br>8. Short stature<br>9. Ethnicity<br>10. Homosexuality | 11. Low parental education (father and mother)<br>12. Low income<br>13. Living in a small town or rural location<br>14. Overcrowding<br>15. Rent accommodations<br>16. Male veterans with a high level of education (12 years+)<br>17. High income hospitalized for depression<br>18. Receiving disability pension because of schizophrenia<br>19. Complicating social factors with bipolar disorder |
| Mental health/ psychiatric illness | 1. Alcohol and/or drug use/ dependence<br>2. Diagnosis of depression<br>3. Any psychiatric disorder diagnosis<br>4. Personality disorder diagnosis<br>5. Anxiety diagnosis<br>6. Schizophrenia diagnosis<br>7. Bipolar disorder diagnosis<br>8. Neurotic disorder diagnosis | 9. Affective episodes in previous year<br>10. Psychiatric inpatient care<br>11. Any mood disorder diagnosis in men who recently had a baby (30–60 days postpartum)<br>12. PTSD in veterans<br>13. Taking medication for psychiatric problems<br>14. Alcohol- related and substance-related mental illness<br>15. Bipolar disorder and a comorbid eating disorder<br>16. Current recurrent psychotic syndrome following a suicide attempt |
| Characteristics of suicidal behavior | 1. History of previous suicide attempt<br>2. Disclosing intent to harm oneself<br>3. Choice of lethal or high-risk method | |

*Data from* Richardson, Robb, & O'Connor.[2]

**Table 2**
**Personal factors contributing to increased suicide risk in men**

| Risk Subgroup | Risk Factors | |
|---|---|---|
| Physical health/illness | 1. Being underweight<br>2. Being obese<br>3. Smoking history<br>4. Cancer diagnosis<br>5. Diabetes diagnosis<br>6. Any type of pain<br>7. Comorbidities (3–4 total) | 8. Poor self-rated health<br>9. Hypertension diagnosis<br>10. Multiple sclerosis diagnosis<br>11. Somatic disorders<br>12. Having activity limitations<br>13. Unexplained weight loss |
| Negative life events/trauma | 1. Adverse childhood experiences<br>2. Bereavement<br>3. Involvement in criminal activity<br>4. Low control at work<br>5. Patient with bipolar disorder who endorsed expressing violent behavior<br>6. Parental psychotic or affective disorder | 7. Stressful life events in the past 6 months<br>8. Childhood sexual victimization<br>9. Aggressive behavior when angry<br>10. Conduct problems in school<br>11. Social isolation as a child |
| Psychological factors | 1. Low IQ<br>2. Poor emotional control<br>3. Externalizing problems<br>4. Poor psychological function capability/poor psychological capability<br>5. Angry behavior when discharged from an inpatient psychiatric facility<br>6. Paranoid states | |

*Data from* Richardson, Robb, & O'Connor.[2]

## PRIMARY CARE CLINICAL APPROACH
### Sociodemographic Characteristics

Many of the risk factors that would contribute to increased suicidality from a sociodemographic stance can be captured on a new patient intake using the electronic health record (EHR) system.[5,29,30] The literature supports the reliability and validity of EHR systems as a useful tool in helping to screen for and predict suicidality based on machine learning and predictive modeling based on assessment data.[5,29–31] Taking a look at some of the risk factors in **Table 1**, information such as marital/relationship status, employment status, living accommodations, home location, veteran status, educational level, income, sexual preference, and ethnicity should be part of new patient documentation. This information alone, aside from what can be gleaned from a thorough history and physical examination (stature, disability status, and comorbidities) can account for most of the information most needed to assess for suicidality.

Use of a screening tool (eg, Patient Health Questionnaire or Suicide Behaviors Questionnaire), if indicated, may help provide a snapshot for suicide risk, as a study shows, that one-half of those who died from suicide sought health care services in the month before their death, and 24% had received services for their mental health.[32,33] Though the US Preventive Services Task Force (USPSTF) does not support the universal screening of all patients for suicide, inclusion of multifactorial suicide risk screens into practice, where appropriate, and inclusion of a universal screening process, could be beneficial.[32,33] Working to improve one's suicide literacy as a nursing professional can not only help with increased provision of quality care aimed at suicide reduction but assist in promoting self-care through the reduction of stigma associated with seeking help.[34–36]

### Mental Health/Psychiatric Illness

The literature supports that most suicides are connected to mental illness/psychiatric disorders, with a suggested link of over 90% when tied to suicide deaths.[20,37–40] Overcoming the stigma associated with mental illness and seeking care (help-seeking behavior) can be difficult for men, and recognizing suicidal ideation in the near-term danger zone can be difficult for care providers.[41,42] A complete past medical history, to include family and social history, can lay the foundation for self-harm prevention and detection, and although risk factors may change throughout the phases of one's life, the strength of association with suicide to psychiatric illness means there will opportunities to intervene for the good of the patient.[43–45] Routine screening and appropriate diagnosis and treatment, be it medical management or psychotherapy, will help determine how severe the risk is of suicide. A good rapport and an open line of communication with patients can increase the chances of disclosure of suicidal ideation, which is vital to suicide prevention.[37,46]

As any diagnosed psychiatric disorder can be a risk factor for suicide, strict attention should be given to comorbid psychiatric disorders, with appropriate referrals provided if the complexity of psychiatric management is outside of one's professional scope.[2,20,24,37] Accurate diagnosis and evidence-based treatment (pharmacological or psychological), along with the use of a suicide prediction tool like the Columbia Suicide Severity Rating Scale (C-SSRS) or the Beck Depression Inventory, will help monitor and manage care proactively so as to follow the National Strategy for Suicide Prevention recommendations.[44,47–49] Substance abuse or dependence, alone, or coupled with another mental health concern, should be addressed with appropriate education and treatment, especially if pharmacologic therapy is used for care. Whether it be anxiety, post-traumatic stress disorder (PTSD), schizophrenia, unipolar or bipolar depression, and/or other mood disorder complicating the clinical picture, regular follow-up visits with inquiry into suicidal intent, and an effort to help ensure a safe home environment for the patient can be part of a comprehensive approach.[44]

### Characteristics of Suicidal Behavior

The history of suicide attempt(s), especially within the last 12 months, is a significant independent risk factor for suicide.[50,51] It is important given the underdisclosing of intent to self-harm that additional attention is given to monitoring and predicting future ideations and actions.[2,20,50,51] Although the disclosure of intent to self-harm is a major risk factor for suicide, reliance upon accurate disclosure from the patient can become concerning, as it may be purposefully concealed.[20,52] Assessment of other risk factors and inquiry into warning signs can assist in making up for the decreased reliability of intent disclosure.[11,52] The chosen method used for suicide matters greatly with regard to the likelihood of being completed.[19,53]

With men more likely to use firearms or hanging as a means for suicide as opposed to poisoning or drowning, the lethality or higher-risk methodology contributes to the gender paradox, and inquiry must be made as to planning and limiting access to highly lethal means.[2,19,53,54]

### Physical Health/Illness

A man's physical health or lack thereof (including multiple comorbidities) has a notable impact on suicidality.[55–57] This is suspected to be due to the impact of physical illness on psychological well-being.[56,57] Increased limitations in daily activity, or functional disability, secondary to or independent from other serious illnesses such as cancer and multiple sclerosis, increase risk of suicide.[58,59] The self-perception of poor health can impact the risk of suicide, as can pain, diabetes, hypertension, somatic disorders, being obese, or being underweight.[2] Knowing the factors linked to increased suicide risk can change the course of care, in that primary care of conditions can address many physical illnesses without additional psychiatric care. This allows closer oversight and interaction, which, as conditions potentially improve, could improve self-rated health.

### Negative Life Events/Trauma

Negative life events or previous trauma can significantly impact mental health and are a predictor of depressive symptoms and hopelessness.[60–62] Linked to anxiety, poor executive function, impulsivity, and ruminative thinking, childhood trauma contributes to suicidal ideation.[63,64] The onset of mental illness is associated with negative life events or previous trauma.[65] Though nothing can be done to change the past when caring for patients, ensuring that they receive proper counseling and behavioral therapy to confront and work through their past trauma is vital to reducing suicide risk. Providing patient education on coping strategies to best minimize aggressive responses and violent behavior, while providing active encouragement to avoid criminal activity, can address several of the risk factors. Adverse experiences at work coupled with psychosocial job stressors constitute a risk factor suicide for men in the workplace, as they contribute to the development of anxiety and depression.[66,67]

### Psychological Factors

Having poor emotional control, referred to as neuroticism, and lower baseline intelligence are associated with increase suicide risk.[68] With directed effort by a clinician, education can be provided to improve self-care, and coping strategies can be reinforced that could negate much of the associated risk.[68] Externalizing or disruptive behaviors include impulsivity, risk-taking behaviors, and the misuse of substances, often with an aggressive or inattentive stance; these behaviors can include being disobedient and even criminal.[69,70] Seeking to address the specific type disruptive behavior via counseling or with pharmacologic treatment, if indicated, can curtail the potential for outbursts. Seeking to address and improve poor functional capacity psychologically and proper evaluation of disability or limitation would signal effectively what psychosocial and pharmacologic interventions would be pursued and assessed periodically for effect.[71] The propensity for anger and aggressive behavior in a patient who has been discharged from an inpatient psychiatric facility would involve engaging the patient to assess what solutions exist to the perceived issue and to ensure further inpatient care is not warranted. Lastly, paranoid or persecutorial states require a rapid response to care given their markedly elevated risk of suicide. If unfamiliar with the screening devices used or uncomfortable with the pharmacologic regimen, expedited referral to a psychiatric professional is warranted.[72]

## GENDER-SENSITIZED SCREENING

With the diagnosis of any psychiatric disorder being such a strong independent risk factor for suicide, assessment of men for a more specific clinical phenotype of such disorders may be worth exploring.[70] A diagnosis of depression, for example, is a well-researched risk factor, but if males present with a different symptomatology from their female counterparts, like externalizing symptoms, their depressive syndrome may not register as well on screening tools like the PHQ-9.[70,73] This being said, an accurate assessment of risk and screening for depression may need to be gender-sensitized like the Gender-Sensitive Depression Screening (GSDS).[70,74,75] Such screening tools have been created in recent years, but there are far more traditional screening tools for depression and suicidality that may under-report symptoms (**Table 3** for examples). Becoming familiar with the screening tools and increasing suicide literacy, clinicians will be able to select the clinical practice guidelines and tools that best fit their clinical setting (eg, emergency room, primary care, or inpatient psychiatric hospital).

## DISCUSSION

Suicide may be a difficult public health problem to tackle, but given the impact it has on the lives of people worldwide, clinicians owe it to their patients to become more knowledgeable on the complexity of screening, prevention, and treatment to reduce its incidence as much as possible. Having a thorough understanding of the risk factors that are commonly observed and the unique ways men may present clinically better informs the care that can be provided. Reassessing how males may present with mental illness and if that is accurately captured in screening tools is important lest the opportunity to intervene and prevent a suicide attempt is missed. With the stigma of mental illness having the potential to impact help-seeking behaviors, thinking outside the box about recognizing warning signs could make all the difference.[76] Reviewing the heterogeneity of risk factors for suicide in men and women cannot help but shine a light on the need to reevaluate universal screening tools.[32] It is also

**Table 3**
**Traditional and gender-sensitive screening tools for depression and suicidality**

| Gender-Sensitized Screening Tools for Depression | Traditional Screening Tools for Depression | Traditional Screening Tools for Suicidality |
| --- | --- | --- |
| Gotland Male Depression Scale (GMDS)[70,74] | Patient Health Questionnaire (PHQ-9) | Scale for Suicide Ideation |
| Masculine Depression Scale (MDS) | Beck Depression Inventory (BDI) | Beck's Suicide Intent Scale |
| Male Depression Risk Scale (MDRS) | Beck Depression Inventory Revision (BDI-II) | Columbia Suicide Severity Rating Scale (C-SSRS) |
| Gender-Sensitive Depression Screening (GSDS) | Center for Epidemiologic Studies Depression Scale (CES-D) | Army STARRS suicide prediction tool |
| | Montgomery-Åsberg Depression Rating Scale (MADRS) | Ask Suicide-Screening Questions (ASQ) |
| | Quick Inventory of Depressive Symptomatology-Self-Report (QIDS-SR) | Patient Safety Screener (PSS-3) |
| | Geriatric Depression Scale (GDS) | OxMIS tool |
| | | Suicide Assessment Five-step Evaluation and Triage (SAFE-T) |
| | | Suicide Behaviors Questionnaire-Revised (SBQ-R |

important to remember that suicidal ideation that is self-reported is not the only relevant factor in assessment, and further insight is needed to better address the unique needs of men with regards to suicide.[32] Further research into the difference of presenting symptoms and risk factors with respect to gender for mental illness and suicide is clearly needed. A deeper dive into the screening tactics, preventative measures, and available treatment regimens offers a lot of future research opportunity.

## SUMMARY

It is important to review the relevant research regarding risk factors for suicidal behaviors in men given the human costs involved. Shared risk factors for suicide are certain to exist among the genders but where they differ could help understand why the gender paradox exists and hopefully reduce the death rate for men. With men more likely to die from suicide attempts than women, it is necessary to evaluate why that is and how to pursue change in fixing it. When subdivided, the risk factors are easier to assess and can be better understood. Health care providers should help patients understand there is care for their underlying mental health problems that could help to prevent the suicidal ideations and behaviors before they begin.

There ought be no shame is speaking up and seeking care for a psychiatric illness. Looking at available screening tools, clinical practice guidelines, and systematic reviews can help one coordinate an action plan and build out an EHR system better equipped to recognize unfamiliar clinical presentations that deviate from universal screening aids.

## CLINICS CARE POINTS

- Become familiar with the risk factors of suicidality in men and the gender differences in clinical symptomatology. Screening tools may not capture them all.
- Use the resources available (eg, EHR, self-report, or screening tools) to build a proactive, multifactorial screening process for suicidal ideation and behavior.
- Any patient with the past medical history of a diagnosed psychiatric illness should be screened for suicide risk.
- Ask the tough questions... Inquire about past suicide attempts and current or former plans.

## DISCLOSURE

The author has no material financial interests or potential conflicts to disclose related to the information described in this article.

## REFERENCES

1. Knipe D, Padmanathan P, Newton-Howes G, et al. Suicide and self-harm. Lancet 2022;399(10338):1903–16.
2. Richardson C, Robb KA, O'Connor RC. A systematic review of suicidal behaviour in men: a narrative synthesis of risk factors. Soc Sci Med 2021;276:113831.
3. Naghavi M. Global Burden of Disease Self-Harm Collaborators. Global, regional, and national burden of suicide mortality 1990 to 2016: systematic analysis for the Global Burden of Disease Study 2016. BMJ 2019;364:l94.
4. National Institute of Mental Health. Suicide. Updated June, 2022. Available at: https://www.nimh.nih.gov/health/statistics/suicide. Accessed January 15, 2023.

5. Nock MK, Millner AJ, Ross EL, et al. Prediction of suicide attempts using clinician assessment, patient self-report, and electronic health records. JAMA Netw Open 2022;5(1):e2144373.

6. Klonsky ED, May AM, Saffer BY. Suicide, suicide attempts, and suicidal ideation. Annu Rev Clin Psychol 2016;12:307–30.

7. Borders A. Rumination and dysregulated behaviors. In: Borders A, editor. Rumination and related constructs: causes, consequences, and treatment of thinking too much. Cambridge, MA: Academic Press; 2020. p. 101–34.

8. Sher L, Oquendo MA. Suicide: an overview for clinicians. Med Clin North Am 2023;107(1):119–30.

9. Schneider RA, Chen SY, Lungu A, et al. Treating suicidal ideation in the context of depression. BMC Psychiatr 2020;20(1):497.

10. Hunt T, Wilson CJ, Caputi P, et al. Signs of current suicidality in men: a systematic review. PLoS One 2017;12(3):e0174675.

11. Bagge CL, Littlefield AK, Wiegand TJ, et al. A controlled examination of acute warning signs for suicide attempts among hospitalized patients. Psychol Med 2022;1–9. https://doi.org/10.1017/S0033291721004712.

12. Howarth E, Johnson J. Comprehensive and clinically useful: review of risk factors for suicidal behaviour in men. Evid Based Nurs 2022;25(3):103.

13. World Health Organization. Suicide. Updated June 17, 2021. Available at: https://www.who.int/news-room/fact-sheets/detail/suicide. Accessed January 15, 2023.

14. World Health Organization. Suicide worldwide in 2019: global health estimates. Updated June 16, 2021. Available at: https://www.who.int/publications/i/item/9789240026643. Accessed January 15, 2023.

15. Centers for Disease Control & Prevention. Underlying cause of death, 2018-2021, single race results. Updated January 17, 2023. Available at: https://wonder.cdc.gov/controller/saved/D158/D321F126. Accessed January 20, 2023.

16. Garnett MF, Curtin SC, Stone DM. Suicide mortality in the United States, 2000–2020. NCHS data brief, no 433. Hyattsville, MD: National Center for Health Statistics; 2022. https://doi.org/10.15620/cdc:114217.

17. Ehlman DC, Yard E, Stone DM, et al. Changes in suicide rates - United States, 2019 and 2020. MMWR Morb Mortal Wkly Rep 2022;71(8):306–12.

18. Garnett MF, Curtin SC, Stone DM. Suicide mortality in the United States, 2000-2020. NCHS Data Brief 2022;(433):1–8.

19. Berardelli I, Rogante E, Sarubbi S, et al. Is lethality different between males and females? Clinical and gender differences in inpatient suicide attempters. Int J Environ Res Public Health 2022;19(20):13309.

20. Bachmann S. Epidemiology of suicide and the psychiatric perspective. Int J Environ Res Public Health 2018;15(7):1425.

21. Bernert RA, Hom MA, Roberts LW. A review of multidisciplinary clinical practice guidelines in suicide prevention: toward an emerging standard in suicide risk assessment and management, training and practice. Acad Psychiatry 2014;38(5):585–92.

22. Zalsman G, Hawton K, Wasserman D, et al. Suicide prevention strategies revisited: 10-year systematic review. Lancet Psychiatr 2016;3(7):646–59.

23. Favril L, Yu R, Uyar A, et al. Risk factors for suicide in adults: systematic review and meta-analysis of psychological autopsy studies. Evid Based Ment Health 2022;25(4):148–55.

24. Cavanagh JT, Carson AJ, Sharpe M, et al. Psychological autopsy studies of suicide: a systematic review. Psychol Med 2003;33(3):395–405, published correction appears in Psychol Med. 2003 Jul;33(5):947.

25. INSERM Collective Expertise Centre. Suicide: psychological autopsy, a research tool for prevention. Paris (FR): Institut national de la Santé et de la recherche Médicale; 2005.

26. Jacobs D, Klein-Benheim M. The psychological autopsy: a useful tool for determining proximate causation in suicide cases. Bull Am Acad Psychiatry Law 1995;23(2):165–82.

27. Griffin L, Hosking W, Gill PR, et al. The gender paradox: understanding the role of masculinity in suicidal ideation. Am J Men's Health 2022;16(5). https://doi.org/10.1177/15579883221123853. 15579883221123853.

28. Janca E, Keen C, Willoughby M, et al. Sex differences in suicide, suicidal ideation, and self-harm after release from incarceration: a systematic review and meta-analysis. Soc Psychiatry Psychiatr Epidemiol 2023;58(3):355–71.

29. Barak-Corren Y, Castro VM, Nock MK, et al. Validation of an electronic health record-based suicide risk prediction modeling approach across multiple health care systems. JAMA Netw Open 2020;3(3):e201262.

30. Barak-Corren Y, Castro VM, Javitt S, et al. Predicting suicidal behavior from longitudinal electronic health records. Am J Psychiatry 2017;174(2):154–62.

31. Walker RL, Shortreed SM, Ziebell RA, et al. Evaluation of electronic health record-based suicide risk prediction models on contemporary data. Appl Clin Inform 2021;12(4):778–87.

32. King CA, Horwitz A, Czyz E, et al. Suicide Risk screening in healthcare settings: identifying males and females at risk. J Clin Psychol Med Settings 2017; 24(1):8–20.

33. Dillon EC, Huang Q, Deng S, et al. Implementing universal suicide screening in a large healthcare system's hospitals: rates of screening, suicide risk, and documentation of subsequent psychiatric care. Transl Behav Med 2023;ibac117. https://doi.org/10.1093/tbm/ibac117, published online ahead of print, 2023 Jan 24.

34. Cruwys T, An S, Chang MX, et al. Suicide literacy predicts the provision of more appropriate support to people experiencing psychological distress. Psychiatry Res 2018;264:96–103.

35. Karakaya D, Özparlak A, Önder M. Suicide literacy in nurses: a cross-sectional study. J Clin Nurs 2023;32(1–2):115–25.

36. Oliffe JL, Hannan-Leith MN, Ogrodniczuk JS, et al. Men's depression and suicide literacy: a nationally representative Canadian survey. J Ment Health 2016;25(6): 520–6.

37. Brådvik L. Suicide risk and mental disorders. Int J Environ Res Public Health 2018;15(9):2028.

38. Robins E, Murphy GE, Wilkinson RH, Jr, et al. Some clinical considerations in the prevention of suicide based on a study of 134 successful suicides. Am J Public Health Nation's Health 1959;49:888–99.

39. Wasserman D, Carli V, Iosue M, et al. Suicide prevention in psychiatric patients. Asia Pac Psychiatry 2021;13(3):e12450.

40. Knipe D, Williams AJ, Hannam-Swain S, et al. Psychiatric morbidity and suicidal behaviour in low- and middle-income countries: a systematic review and meta-analysis. PLoS Med 2019;16(10):e1002905.

41. Calear AL, Batterham PJ, Christensen H. Predictors of help-seeking for suicidal ideation in the community: risks and opportunities for public suicide prevention campaigns. Psychiatry Res 2014;219(3):525–30.

42. Berman AL. Risk factors proximate to suicide and suicide risk assessment in the context of denied suicide ideation. Suicide Life Threat Behav 2018;48(3):340–52.

43. Yeh HH, Westphal J, Hu Y, et al. Diagnosed mental health conditions and risk of suicide mortality. Psychiatr Serv 2019;70(9):750–7.
44. Fazel S, Runeson B. Suicide. N Engl J Med 2020;382(3):266–74, published correction appears in N Engl J Med. 2020 Mar 12;382(11):1078.
45. Troya MI, Babatunde O, Polidano K, et al. Self-harm in older adults: systematic review. Br J Psychiatry 2019;214(4):186–200.
46. Mérelle S, Foppen E, Gilissen R, et al. Characteristics associated with non-disclosure of suicidal ideation in adults. Int J Environ Res Public Health 2018; 15(5):943.
47. Iskander JK, Crosby AE. Implementing the national suicide prevention strategy: time for action to flatten the curve. Prev Med 2021;152(Pt 1):106734.
48. Runeson B, Odeberg J, Pettersson A, et al. Instruments for the assessment of suicide risk: a systematic review evaluating the certainty of the evidence. PLoS One 2017;12(7):e0180292.
49. Lindh ÅU, Waern M, Beckman K, et al. Short term risk of non-fatal and fatal suicidal behaviours: the predictve validity of the Columbia-Suicide Severity Rating Scale in a Swedish adult psychiatric population with a recent episode of self-harm. BMC Psychiatr 2018;18(1):319.
50. Demesmaeker A, Chazard E, Hoang A, et al. Suicide mortality after a nonfatal suicide attempt: a systematic review and meta-analysis. Aust N Z J Psychiatry 2022; 56(6):603–16.
51. Reutfors J, Andersson TM, Tanskanen A, et al. Risk factors for suicide and suicide attempts among patients with treatment-resistant depression: nested case-control study. Arch Suicide Res 2021;25(3):424–38.
52. Rogers ML, Bloch-Elkouby S, Galynker I. Differential disclosure of suicidal intent to clinicians versus researchers: associations with concurrent suicide crisis syndrome and prospective suicidal ideation and attempts. Psychiatry Res 2022;312: 114522.
53. Cai Z, Junus A, Chang Q, et al. The lethality of suicide methods: a systematic review and meta-analysis. J Affect Disord 2022;300:121–9.
54. Cibis A, Mergl R, Bramesfeld A, et al. Preference of lethal methods is not the only cause for higher suicide rates in males. J Affect Disord 2012;136(1–2):9–16.
55. Ahmedani BK, Peterson EL, Hu Y, et al. Major physical health conditions and risk of suicide. Am J Prev Med 2017;53(3):308–15.
56. Onyeka IN, Maguire A, Ross E, et al. Does physical ill-health increase the risk of suicide? A census-based follow-up study of over 1 million people. Epidemiol Psychiatr Sci 2020;29:e140.
57. Nafilyan V, Morgan J, Mais D, et al. Risk of suicide after diagnosis of severe physical health conditions: a retrospective cohort study of 47 million people. Lancet Reg Health Eur 2022;25:100562.
58. Phillips JA, Hempstead K. The role of context in shaping the relationship between physical health and suicide over the life course. SSM Popul Health 2022;17: 101059.
59. Fässberg MM, Cheung G, Canetto SS, et al. A systematic review of physical illness, functional disability, and suicidal behaviour among older adults. Aging Ment Health 2016;20(2):166–94.
60. Chen T, Roberts K. Negative life events and suicide in the national violent death reporting system. Arch Suicide Res 2021;25(2):238–52.
61. Ji L, Chen C, Hou B, et al. A study of negative life events driven depressive symptoms and academic engagement in Chinese college students. Sci Rep 2021; 11(1):17160.

62. Hirsch JK, Hall BB, Wise HA, et al. Negative life events and suicide risk in college students: conditional indirect effects of hopelessness and self-compassion. J Am Coll Health 2021;69(5):546–53.

63. Rogerson O, Baguley T, O'Connor DB. Childhood trauma and suicide. Crisis 2022. https://doi.org/10.1027/0227-5910/a000886 [published online ahead of print, 2022 Dec 20].

64. Valderrama J, Macrynikola N, Miranda R. Early life trauma, suicide ideation, and suicide attempts: the role of rumination and impulsivity. Arch Suicide Res 2022; 26(2):731–47.

65. Fuse-Nagase Y, Marutani T, Watanabe K, et al. Negative life events are associated with risk of mental illness among Japanese university students. Psychiatry and Clinical Neurosciences Reports 2023;2. https://doi.org/10.1002/pcn5.78.

66. Milner A, Spittal MJ, Pirkis J, et al. Low control and high demands at work as risk factors for suicide: an australian national population-level case-control study. Psychosom Med 2017;79(3):358–64.

67. Griffin JM, Fuhrer R, Stansfeld SA, et al. The importance of low control at work and home on depression and anxiety: do these effects vary by gender and social class? Soc Sci Med 2002;54(5):783–98.

68. Hansson Bittár N, Falkstedt D, Sörberg Wallin A. How intelligence and emotional control are related to suicidal behavior across the life course - a register-based study with 38-year follow-up. Psychol Med 2020;50(13):2265–71.

69. Soto-Sanz V, Castellví P, Piqueras JA, et al. Internalizing and externalizing symptoms and suicidal behaviour in young people: a systematic review and meta-analysis of longitudinal studies. Acta Psychiatr Scand 2019;140(1):5–19.

70. Oliffe JL, Rossnagel E, Seidler ZE, et al. Men's depression and suicide. Curr Psychiatry Rep 2019;21(10):103.

71. Patterson TL, Mausbach BT. Measurement of functional capacity: a new approach to understanding functional differences and real-world behavioral adaptation in those with mental illness. Annu Rev Clin Psychol 2010;6:139–54.

72. Freeman D, Bold E, Chadwick E, et al. Suicidal ideation and behaviour in patients with persecutory delusions: prevalence, symptom associations, and psychological correlates. Compr Psychiatry 2019;93:41–7.

73. Rutz W, Wålinder J, Von Knorring L, et al. Prevention of depression and suicide by education and medication: impact on male suicidality. An update from the Gotland Study. Int J Psychiatry Clin Pract 1997;1(1):39–46.

74. Sigurdsson B, Palsson SP, Aevarsson O, et al. Validity of Gotland Male Depression Scale for male depression in a community study: the Sudurnesjamenn Study. J Affect Disord 2015;173:81–9.

75. Streb J, Ruppel E, Möller-Leimkühler AM, et al. Gender-specific differences in depressive behavior among forensic psychiatric patients. Front Psychol 2021; 12:639191.

76. Schomerus G, Angermeyer MC. Stigma and its impact on help-seeking for mental disorders: what do we know? Epidemiol Psichiatr Soc 2008;17(1):31–7.

# The Role of Testosterone Therapy in Men's Health

Blake K. Smith, MSN, BSN, BS, RN[a,b,c],
Michael Ward, MSN, APRN, AGACNP-BC[d],*

## KEYWORDS

- Low T • Testosterone • Men's health • Testosterone replacement therapy

## KEY POINTS

- It is essential to understand thorough, efficient, and cost-effective assessment and diagnosis of low testosterone.
- Low testosterone can manifest based on comorbid conditions or contribute to other disorders/conditions if not treated.
- There is a continuation of the inconsistency of standardization of guidelines around the globe on best practices for low testosterone treatment.
- To achieve the best treatment outcomes, the provider must consider laboratory assays and the presentation of signs and symptoms.

## INTRODUCTION

Charles Édouard Brown-Séquard injected himself with a mixture containing liquid extracted from the testicles of dogs or guinea pigs in 1889 (Video 1). The therapy was injected 10 times over 3 weeks. Brown-Séquard observed physical changes: an increase in his forearm flexor strength, a more forceful urinary stream, the ability to defecate more efficiently, and a subjective improvement in his cognitive abilities. The once-proclaimed "Elixir of Life," *testosterone* (T), has many well-studied anabolic, metabolic, and developmental properties that affect target organs in men and women. The potential uses of this compound prompted several teams of biochemists to race for isolation of the testicular hormone in the early twentieth century.[1] The surge of athletes hoping to benefit from the anabolic effects of T began in the first half of the twentieth century. It was not until researchers controlled for exercise routines and protein intake that it was identified that testosterone leads to increases in strength, fat-free

[a] American Association for Men in Nursing, Wisconsin Rapids, WI, USA; [b] Clinical Documentation Sr. Analyst, Enterprise Applications, Nebraska Medicine, Omaha, NE, USA; [c] Accelerated Program Student Success Coach, School of Nursing, Nebraska Methodist College, Omaha, NE, USA; [d] Critical Care Nurse Practitioner, Cardiovascular ICU, Medical ICU, Texas Health Huguley Hospital, 11801 South Freeway, Burleson, TX 76028, USA
* Corresponding author. 214 NE Wilshire Boulevard, Burleson, TX 76028.
*E-mail address:* Brandonw.rn@gmail.com

Nurs Clin N Am 58 (2023) 525–539
https://doi.org/10.1016/j.cnur.2023.07.001
0029-6465/23/© 2023 Elsevier Inc. All rights reserved.
nursing.theclinics.com

mass, and overall muscle mass in exercising men.[2] *Testosterone replacement therapy* (TTh), as it has become known, has proved to be an effective treatment strategy for improving the quality of life for hypogonadal men around the globe.

Low levels of circulating serum T characterize *hypogonadism* due to interference or malfunction of the hypothalamic-pituitary-gonadal axis (HPGA). It is estimated to affect 2 to 4 million men annually in North America alone. An estimated 1 in 10 men older than 60 years has a *testosterone deficiency* (TD) and 1 in 3 has diabetes.[3] By 2025, an estimated 6.5 million American men will be affected.[4]

T is a pleiotropic hormone that plays an essential role in the human body. Through its conversion to estrogen, T affects bone health and density. Male hypogonadism is the clinical condition representing symptoms and gonadal dysfunction of Leydig cells, resulting in decreased T, Sertoli cell/germ cells, and decreased sperm production.[5] There has been a renewed interest recently in the systemic role of T in pain, well-being, and cardiovascular function in both women and men.[2]

Therapeutic T levels are linked to improved sexual function, physical performance, strength, lean body mass, and cognitive function and have some cardiovascular benefits.[6,7] Low T levels can lead to sarcopenia, increased adiposity, fatigue, lack of motivation, cardiovascular diseases, cancer, and all-cause mortality.[4,8] Androgen deficiency signs and symptoms take time to manifest clinically in adolescents and young men, given the numerous pathways within the HPGA and reduced efficiency changes to hormonal levels.[5] Experts have debated using TTh in men who might benefit from replacing declining hormone levels.[2] With the recent prolongation of life expectancy, especially in men, the question concerning T replacement in older men has become more important.[9]

## Considerations of Testosterone

### Testosterone production

Androgen synthesis in the gonads of men and women is regulated by the secretion of gonadotropin-releasing hormone (GnRH) from the hypothalamus, releasing luteinizing hormone (LH) and follicle-stimulating hormone (FSH) from the pituitary gland.[2] The HPGA plays a significant role in male hormonal balance maturation, development, and sustainability. The pulsatile secretion of GnRH by the hypothalamus stimulates LH and FSH production and secretion by the anterior pituitary gland. LH stimulates T production from the interstitial Leydig cells of the testes. Male internal and external reproductive organ development requires T production, resulting in the differentiation of secondary human sexual characteristics. FSH, in turn, sustains testicular function via Sertoli cells through spermatogenesis.[10] Ninety-five percent of the synthesis of serum T in men is produced by the Leydig cells of the testis under the influence of LH secreted from the pituitary gland.[5] Evidence from genetic studies of fetal testicular tissue has shown that adrenocorticotropic hormone can stimulate fetal Leydig cells to produce steroids, reinforcing the link between adrenal and testicular tissue.[2]

Dehydroepiandrosterone (DHEA) and DHEA-S are prohormone substrates for forming potent androgens such as T and dihydrotestosterone (DHT) by peripheral conversion. Free T and DHT then bind the intracellular androgen receptor, enabling the complex to bind DNA regions and exert androgenic effects.[2] T can also be converted to estrogen via aromatase, a cytochrome P450 enzyme family member, in target areas, including neural tissue, adipose, liver, and bone. In men, estrogen from this reaction is essential for the maturation of sperm and libido maintenance.[11] Albumin-bound T is also biologically active, given the low affinity of T for the protein.[2]

### Measuring testosterone

The diagnosis of TD requires the presence of characteristic symptoms and signs in combination with decreased serum concentration of T.[12] Although sensitive, screening questionnaires or structured interviews on male symptomatic TD have low specificity.[13] Morley and colleagues compared the most used questionnaires in 148 men using bioavailable testosterone to diagnose TD. They found the sensitivity to be 97% for the ADAM (Androgen Deficiency in the Aging Male questionnaire), 83% for the AMS (Aging Male's Symptoms scale), and 60% for the MMAS (Massachusetts Male Aging Study questionnaire). Specificity was 30% for the ADAM, 59% for the MMAS, and 39% for the AMS.[14] Although other extensive face-to-face comparisons are lacking, more recently, a large systematic review including 40 studies concluded that a specific structured interview, ANDROTEST, for detecting hypogonadism-related symptoms and signs, showed both the most favorable positive and negative likelihood ratio for detecting low T.[13] A 12-item version of the interview (ANDROTEST) had a sensitivity and specificity of 68% and 65% in detecting low total T ($<10.4$ nmol/L) and 71% and 65% in the screening for low free T ($<37$ pmol/L).[15] Given this specificity compared with the ADAM questionnaire, the structured interview hypogonadism screening questionnaires, including the ANDROTEST, may not be as economic and efficient as the ADAM questionnaire as a first-line screening test for hypogonadism.[16] **Fig. 1** is an example of the ADAM Questionnaire developed by Saint Louis University in 2000.

The expected morning T range for men is between 300 and 1000 ng/dL, and *hypogonadism* is defined as a total T less than 300 ng/dL by the Endocrine Society clinical practice guidelines.[17,18] Threshold, along with various others defining low total T set from 250 to 300 ng/dL by other societies such as the American Urological Association, have been established regardless of age following many large-scale population studies.[10] T secretion follows a circadian rhythm in young and aging men, with the highest levels generally occurring in the early morning; therefore, it is recommended that blood samples for T should ideally be drawn in the morning to assess patients'

**Questions Used as Part of the Saint Louis University ADAM Questionnaire**

1. Do you have a decrease in libido (sex drive)?

2. Do you have a lack of energy?

3. Do you have a decrease in strength and/or endurance?

4. Have you lost height?

5. Have you noticed a decreased "enjoyment of life"?

6. Are you sad and/or grumpy?

7. Are your erections less strong?

8. Have you noted a recent deterioration in your ability to play sports?

9. Are you falling asleep after dinner?

10. Has there been a recent deterioration in your work performance?

NOTE. A positive questionnaire result is defined as a "yes" answer to questions 1 or 7 or any 3 other questions.

**Fig. 1.** Androgen Deficiency in Adult Males (A.D.A.M.) Questionnaire

androgen status properly.[2] Free and albumin-bound T is a relatively accurate measure of a patient's clinical and hormonal composition, more so than total hormone levels.[2] Following confirmation of low serum T levels and concomitant signs and symptoms of hypogonadism, clinicians should use serum LH and FSH in conjunction with T to differentiate between primary and secondary hypogonadism.[5] Measuring T levels is challenging; it is essential to appreciate androgen production and regulation.[2]

T assays play a vital role in the workup and diagnosis of many endocrine disorders. Assays in men are used to diagnose clinical *hypogonadism* in patients with prostate cancer (PCa) treated with GnRH analogues and in children to monitor signs and symptoms of advanced and delayed puberty.[2] Sertoli cell assessment is needed to diagnose *hypogonadism* in prepubertal populations.[5] Clinicians should be cognizant that varying measurements between laboratories may be consequences of the method used rather than a reflection of actual changes in T levels. One proposed solution is to measure free rather than serum T, which can be measured by equilibrium dialysis. Free T passes through a membrane into a dialysate solution in this method, but protein-bound testosterone does not.[2]

### Age/environmental factors

A distinction should be made because *hypogonadism* has been defined more so based on adults, children, and adolescents. If not occurring together in *hypogonadism* as hypoandrogenism (Leydig cell dysfunction), other testicular cell populations, germ cells, or Sertoli cells are considered for possible dysfunction.[5] Approximately 70% of children with *hypogonadism* are misdiagnosed based on serum gonadotropin measurement.[19] Male adolescents may present with few typical signs of adult *hypogonadism*, and biochemical androgen levels must be followed-up in the younger cohorts of men so effective clinical research strategies can be recommended.[5] Diagnosing hypoandrogenism in healthy adolescents can be challenging, as the symptoms correlating with a decreased T level are different than in the elderly population. In a recent study, hypogonadal symptoms in men younger than 40 years were associated with a total T level of less than 400 ng/dL. Of the hypogonadal symptoms evaluated with the Aging Male (ADAM) questionnaire, "lack of energy" seems to be the most acute symptom that predicts a total T level of less than 400 ng/dL in men younger than 40 as opposed to erectile dysfunction and decreased libido, which were more frequent complaints in the elderly population.[20] Symptoms of fatigue and lack of energy may be more specific in the younger adult cohort than sexual symptoms. There is increasing evidence that anti-Mullerian and inhibin B levels can improve the sensitivity and result in earlier diagnosis, ultimately allowing treatment to start at a younger age.[5]

Older men have been known to have had declines in serum T levels for some time. However, researchers disputed whether this process naturally occurred or if it was secondary to concurrent comorbidities and related factors.[2] The age-related decrease in T reflects general age-related cellular degeneration, reduced number of functional Leydig cells, and atherosclerosis of testicular arterioles.[21] Increasing age also brought about gradual decreases in free and total T, with increases in gonadotropins, LH, and FSH.[2] The difference between the decline of total T and free T during aging is an age-related increase in the circulating concentration of sex hormone–binding globulin (SHBG), reducing free T proportion.[22]

In the developing world, several increasing conditions may be shifting the prevalence of *hypogonadism* to a younger age, including diabetes, obesity, and increasing rates of opioid use.[23] With the increasing epidemic of adolescent and young adult obesity and type II diabetes, it is plausible that these conditions, in isolation or tandem, may explain lower-than-average androgen levels in patients aged 20 to 40 years.[5] Opioid-induced androgen deficiency has increased dramatically in the last 10 to 15 years. Sexual dysfunction is reported in 85% of heroin addicts and 81% on a stable methadone maintenance regimen, although this might be due to additional factors.[24] Chronic opioid use disrupts the HPGA creating secondary *hypogonadism*. Opioid receptors μ (MOR), δ (DOR), and κ (KOR) are present in the hypothalamus and the pituitary, with activation leading to a suppressed HPGA and subsequent decrease in serum T within hours of opioid administration.[25] Exposure to several environmental toxins may also contribute to *hypogonadism*, notably Sertoli and germ cell dysfunction. Tobacco smoke contains highly carcinogenic nitrosamines, polycyclic aromatic hydrocarbons (benzopyrene), and volatile organic compounds (benzene).[5] Increased seminal levels of reactive oxygen species from smoking impair sperm function, and data show that nicotine and its metabolites can cross the blood-testis barrier.[26]

### Understanding Hypogonadism

TD occurring during adulthood (ie, late-onset *hypogonadism* [LOH]) is a common condition, representing the main endocrine concern in the aging men.[27] Signs and symptoms of low androgen levels include reduced sexual desire and activity, erectile dysfunction, decreased spontaneous erections, incomplete or delayed sexual development, small testes, gynecomastia, loss of body hair/reduced shaving, subfertility, and reduced bone mass. Less specific symptoms and signs are decreased energy and motivation, reduced physical performance, depressed mood, poor concentration and memory, sleep disturbances, anemia, reduced muscle mass, and increased body fat.[5] The benefits of T concerning mental health, mood, cognition, bone density, and pain control should be considered.[2] Clinicians should consider the overlap of TD and chronic conditions when performing the diagnostic workup for *hypogonadism*.[27]

*Hypogonadism* can result from multifactorial conditions, and finding an ideal therapy cannot be a one-size-fits-all approach.[5] Chronic diseases could impair sexual functioning but do not affect sexual motivation, as TD does. Chronic illnesses and TD can be considered overlapping conditions, often sharing the same phenotype and hormonal alterations.[27] There are weak associations between signs and symptoms and serum T levels in aging men. The unimpressive positive likelihood ratios may be because many symptoms and signs of low T are nonspecific—resulting from other comorbid conditions commonly occurring in older men.[28] The condition of primary testicular dysfunction (lower total and free T and high gonadotropins) and its related symptoms (higher ANDROTEST score) are often present in subjects with chronic morbidities. Because hypogonadal symptoms, including the sexual ones and penile blood flow, are known to be affected by T levels, the relative weight and mutual effect of the Chronic Disease Score and total T on these associations were evaluated.[27] Low T level has implications for metabolic health in both men and women and can be a risk factor because it correlates with metabolic syndrome and all-cause mortality.[29] Men with TD not receiving TTh experience a significant increase in body weight, waist size, and deterioration in glycemic control over time. Being overweight or obese underscores the importance of also considering the risks of untreated TD.[30] Many causes of hypoandrogenism in adolescents may be transient, which will resolve low androgen levels once the underlying condition is improved or resolved. **Fig. 2** lists the known disorders of congenital or acquired means of the testicular (primary *hypogonadism*) or HPGA (secondary *hypogonadism*) conditions leading to androgen deficiency.[10]

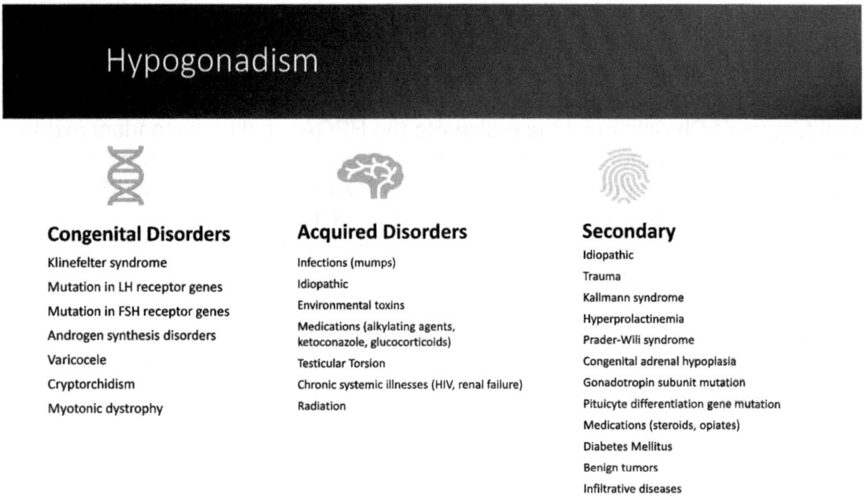

## Hypogonadism

**Congenital Disorders**

Klinefelter syndrome

Mutation in LH receptor genes

Mutation in FSH receptor genes

Androgen synthesis disorders

Varicocele

Cryptorchidism

Myotonic dystrophy

**Acquired Disorders**

Infections (mumps)

Idiopathic

Environmental toxins

Medications (alkylating agents, ketoconazole, glucocorticoids)

Testicular Torsion

Chronic systemic illnesses (HIV, renal failure)

Radiation

**Secondary**

Idiopathic

Trauma

Kallmann syndrome

Hyperprolactinemia

Prader-Wili syndrome

Congenital adrenal hypoplasia

Gonadotropin subunit mutation

Pituicyte differentiation gene mutation

Medications (steroids, opiates)

Diabetes Mellitus

Benign tumors

Infiltrative diseases

**Fig. 2.** Causes of hypogonadism.

## Presentation

### Cardiovascular

The bidirectional role of T and cardiovascular risk is confounding. Some studies claim that TTh increases cardiovascular (CV) risk. Conversely, some studies demonstrate that low T is a CV risk marker, which improves with normalizing T levels after exogenous T administration. This potential CV risk has resulted in the Food and Drug Administration (FDA) releasing a statement about the potential risk associated with TRT.[31] In a large retrospective study with extended follow-up of more than 83,000 male veterans, normalizing T levels after TTh significantly reduced all-cause mortality, myocardial infarction, and stroke.[32] A meta-analysis of observational studies from 1988 to 2017, which consisted of 43,041 men with an average age of 63.5 years, demonstrated that low T in aging men is a marker of CV risk.[33] The lack of adequately powered and long-term randomized control trials on the efficacy and safety of TTh has not helped. However, in 2018 the Testosterone Replacement Therapy for Assessment of Long-term Vascular Events and efficacy ResponSE in hypogonadal men (TRAVERSE) trial became underway. The TRAVERSE study was a double-blind placebo, parallel-group, noninferiority, multicentered controlled trial that randomized approximately 6000 men, ages 45 to 80 years, with baseline serum T less than 300 with hypogonadal symptoms and preexisting CV disease or increased CV risk. The men were randomized to a 1.62% T or placebo gel.[7] The trial was completed on Jan 7, 2023, with results currently being compiled. The required reporting date is Jan 19, 2024.[34]

### Sexual function

Sexual symptoms are the most related explicitly to androgen deficiency.[35] The loss of sexual desire seems as the most genuine hallmark of TD. The presence of a specific association between sexual symptoms and TD is not enough to establish the direction of the relationship; in fact, TD may be responsible for causing the symptoms or the other way around. Symptoms of LOH encompass various domains, including psychological, physical, and sexual disturbances.[27] Studies related to the sexual domain (ie, reduced libido and reduced spontaneous or sexual-related erections) show a syndromic association with TD. Therefore, they could represent a valuable correlate to define a symptomatic LOH.[21] When TD is suspected in men with chronic illnesses, hypoactive sexual desire could help outline an androgen deficiency–related clinical phenotype. Hypoactive sexual desire is more severe in hypogonadal groups irrespective of health status, thus strengthening the concept that sexual desire depends on T with limited influence of chronic conditions.[27]

## Musculoskeletal strength

Lower levels of androgens contributed to decreased lean muscle mass, strength, and size.[36] Sex hormones play a critical role in the maintenance and growth of bone in both men and women. Androgen receptors manifest in chondrocytes in growth plates, osteoblasts, and osteocytes.[2] The most acute effects of testosterone on bone are its aromatization to estradiol, which activates bone $\alpha$ and $\beta$ estrogen receptors, decreasing bone resorption, and increasing bone mineral density.[37] Bone mineral density of the vertebral bone with idiopathic osteoporosis in men increases with TTh. T has also been shown to have associations with vitamin D, which plays a vital role in calcium homeostasis.[2]

The development and progression of chronic diseases are correlated with low T levels and inflammatory biomarkers, but their mechanisms remain poorly understood.[38] A low T level is correlated with a high level of adipokines and inflammation, and T therapy is necessary to restore the physiologic and hormonal levels.[38] Androgen therapy in older men with T deficiency improves physical efficiency and reduces the risk of rehospitalization.[39] Musculoskeletal benefits do not persist after cessation of TTh. Lean body mass decreases within 6 months after discontinuing TTh, although it remains higher than baseline. Strength training in older men with low to normal T levels improved muscle function but not lean body mass. Combined with TTh, strength training led to increased muscle function and mass. In this study, TTh alone did not improve function or mass over the study period.[2]

## Obesity/insulin efficiency

Obesity is a decisive risk factor for TD, which further increases fat accumulation, insulin resistance, and deterioration of glycemic control, creating a vicious circle.[40] The obesity-related decline of T levels is multifactorial.[20] These body composition changes from T have metabolic effects.[41] It can be associated with decreased SHBG or an increased conversion of T to estrogen by peripheral adipose tissue.[20] T and estradiol levels interact to increase muscle mass and decrease body fat.[36] T benefits affect lean muscle mass and body fat.[2] It is well documented that TTh consistently results in a significant reduction in fat mass and an increase in lean mass.[42] This body composition changes from T have metabolic effects.[41] Men with low T are suspectable to increased insulin resistance.[43] Low T is associated with insulin resistance even in young nonobese men.[43] The underlying cause of *hypogonadism* in young obese men is the possibility of a concurrent diagnosis of type 2 diabetes mellitus, which has been increasing at a yearly rate of 4.8% compared with 1.8% for type 1.[44] Seventy-three percent of men with reduced T were overweight or obese, and serum T in men with a body mass index (BMI) greater than 30 kg/m$^2$ was 5 nmol/L lower than those with average weight.[45]

## Cognition/mood

Aging is associated with cognitive decline, including verbal and visual memory, executive function, and spatial ability.[46–48] Aging in men is also associated with reduced serum T, raising the possibility that reduced circulating T concentration may contribute to age-related cognitive decline. Support for this hypothesis comes from studies of clinical conditions that cause low T levels, epidemiological investigations, and small randomized trials showing improved memory with T supplementation. Among psychological traits, depressive symptoms were the most specific to low T, associated with it independently of comorbidities.[27] A meta-analysis explicitly focusing on the effects of TTh on mood found an improvement in T-treated men, which was maintained independently of a chronic condition.[5]

### Prostate cancer

In healthy men, the androgen T and its derivative DHT are essential for cell survival and function of the prostate.[49] Low serum T was associated with a higher risk of poorly differentiated PCa, albeit BMI was not considered in the data analysis.[49] PCa cells exhibit excess activation of the androgen signaling pathway, resulting in the uncontrolled proliferation of tumor cells.[50] Almost all PCa tumors will initially respond to androgen deprivation therapy (ADT). However, with long-term T suppression, some cell populations become refractory, and eliminating T production from the testes is no longer sufficient to suppress tumor cell growth entirely.[51] This growth is called castration-resistant PCa, which an increasing prostate-specific antigen determines in an environment where T levels are castrated. There is increasing evidence that deficient nadir T levels, particularly during the first few months of ADT, and the absence of micro-surges and escapes in T may be associated with improved clinical outcomes, including survival.[52] This low T environment seems to promote the development of a less differentiated, aggressive cancer phenotype.[53]

### Treatment

There is much to consider by both the patient and the provider when initiating TTh. Historically, TTh has been the most used option in treating primary and *secondary hypogonadism*.[54] However, for *secondary hypogonadism*, there are very effective additional treatment options available that have been used off-label for some time. As mentioned previously, *secondary hypogonadism* results in an interruption in T production due to the HPGA. This interruption could include *age-related hypogonadism*, *obesity-related hypogonadism, opioid-induced hypogonadism*, metabolic syndrome, and type 2 diabetes mellitus.[55]

Various formulations of TTh exist, offering options with different pharmacologic profiles, delivery methods, and half-lives. T formulations with shorter half-lives are more consistent with endogenous T production but often result in nonadherence due to the multiple-day dosing.[56] Longer-acting formulations have proved much more feasible for patients, with some preparations only requiring weekly and even monthly administration. One delivery method is implanted under the skin once every 2 to 4 months. However, there are drawbacks to the more prolonged duration preparations. The longer the half-life, the higher the likelihood of adverse effects, for example, impaired sperm parameters.[56]

## DELIVERY METHODS

As mentioned earlier, there are various routes of delivery and formulations available on the market today. Each delivery route brings advantages and disadvantages. In short-acting formulations, the advantage is convenience and painless application. Short-acting delivery methods include intranasal sprays; transdermal applications such as a gel, cream, or patch; and oral formulations in capsules and troches.

*Natesto* intranasal is a nasal spray used daily. Some of the adverse effects associated with its use include mucosal dryness, rhinorrhea, epistaxis, and even upper respiratory tract infections. Although, these adverse reactions occur in less than 9% of those who use them.[56] *Fortesta Gel, AndroGel*, and *Testim Gel* are topical compounds applied under the arm or behind the knee daily. The most common adverse reaction reported was skin irritation.[56] An important consideration with gels and creams is the risk of transference if one should contact another person. *Androderm* patches are transdermal patches applied to the skin daily. Gurayah and colleagues[56] cite a study demonstrating that up to 18.8% of patients who used *Androderm* patches experienced administration site reactions, that is, pruritis and erythema. *Jatenzo* and *Tlando* are daily oral capsules. With *Jatenzo*, elevated hematocrit was higher than all other formulations and resulted in higher blood pressure in a few participants.[56] *Tlando* resulted in elevated levels of prolactin and weight gain.[56]

Long-acting formulations also bring with them their advantages and disadvantages. Longer-acting formulations require fewer administrations throughout the month. These formulations come in the form of injectable T and subcutaneous pellets. Injectable T has been used since the late 1930s and has proved to maintain T levels.[3] The first T injectable was called testosterone propionate. With a half-life of 1 to 2 days, testosterone propionate was discontinued due to other formulations with longer half-lives. Testosterone cypionate and enanthate are the gold standards for injectable TTh. They both have similar half-lives of approximately 8 days. Risks of injectable T include bleeding and discomfort. Testosterone undecanoate is administered every 10 to 12 weeks. Unlike testosterone cypionate and enanthate, testosterone undecanoate must be administered by a health care professional due to its ability to cause microembolism and anaphylaxis.[3] Testosterone cypionate and enanthate can be self-administered at home.

Subcutaneous T pellets are inserted under the skin into the soft tissue every 2 to 4 months. Some providers will insert pellets for up to 6 months. Each subcutaneous pellet contains 75 mg of T. The number of pellets inserted depends on the BMI of the patient. A person with a BMI greater than 25 can have up to 12 pellets inserted. The risks associated with subcutaneous pellets include rejection, injection site infection, hemorrhage, fibrosis, or scarring with prolonged use of T pellets. In addition, if one's laboratory result values do not reflect optimal dosing after insertion, another incision is required to insert additional pellets.

## POTENTIAL ALTERNATIVE USES

Exogenous T has demonstrated many benefits regarding sexual health in men, including enhanced libido and improved erection quality. However, exogenous T is known to interfere with the HPGA, resulting in decreased production of LH and FSH. The following result is testicular atrophy and oligospermia. There is a contraindication for TTh in men who have inclinations of having children soon. However, there are other options available for men in this demographic. Gonadotropins, aromatase inhibitors, and selective estrogen receptor modulators (SERMS) effectively treat secondary hypogonadism while maintaining fertility.[3,8]

Exogenous gonadotropins, similar to human chorionic gonadotropin, stimulate the Leydig cells to produce T because of their similarity to LH and have been effectively used in men with oligospermia or azoospermia.[3] These medications are administered intramuscularly or subcutaneously. Aromatase inhibitors, such as anastrazole, preserve T levels by inhibiting the aromatization of T to estradiol. Aromatase inhibitors can maintain therapeutic T levels without affecting sperm counts. However, over time, these medications can cause deficient estrogen levels, resulting in decreased bone density and increased risk of fractures.

SERMS show the most promise. In addition to maintaining fertility and increasing baseline T levels, SERMs are not shown to cause supratherapeutic T levels.[54]

Clomiphene citrate, also known as Clomid, was introduced in the 1960s for women and is the most widely used SERM for treating *hypogonadism* in men wishing to have children. Ide and colleagues reviewed 5 randomized controlled trials on the use of SERMs for hypogonadal men. In one study, out of 400 men treated with clomiphene citrate for 25.5 months, only 8% reported side effects. The most common side effects were mood changes, blurred vision, breast tenderness, and weight gain. These side effects were a result of elevated estradiol levels. Another study of 46 men treated for more than 12 months reported no side effects. Despite not being FDA approved for use in men or patients with *hypogonadism*, the extensively researched use of this "off-label" indication proves to effectively treat men for this purpose.[8] However, despite its known safety and efficacy, more research is needed.

Clomiphene citrate consists of 2 isomers, enclomiphene, the trans-isomer, and zuclomiphene, the cis-isomer. Enclomiphene is an estrogen antagonist, whereas zuclomiphene is an estrogen agonist. This distinction is why clomiphene citrate has caused elevated estradiol levels in some.[57] Enclomiphene is more potent than clomiphene, causing more significant increases in serum T levels while, in some studies, significantly raising sperm counts.[57] Enclomiphene is well tolerated and causes mild side effects in a low percentage of those studied. The most concerning adverse effect of SERMs is the increased risk of venous thromboembolism. According to Earl and Kim,[57] this incidence has been very low. Other side effects include headache 3.3%, nausea 2.1%, diarrhea 1.9%, nasopharyngitis 1,7%, hot flashes 1.7%, arthralgia 1.2%, and dizziness 1%.[57] Enclomiphene demonstrates significant effectiveness in raising baseline T levels while preserving fertility and without raising estrogen levels. However, the FDA did not approve the drug because the lack of data indicates improvement in clinical symptoms; this is an area of research that should be explored. Much more could be discussed here, but it is beyond the scope of this article.

## REPLACEMENT THERAPY VERSUS OPTIMIZATION

*TTh is* a T treatment regimen that results in therapeutic serum T levels. T optimization refers to optimizing T levels for maximum benefit and well-being without achieving supratherapeutic levels well above the established reference ranges. The US serum T reference ranges from 264 to 916 ng/dL for healthy, nonobese men. Many providers will not initiate T treatment if the total serum T is less than 264, despite having symptoms consistent with *hypogonadism*.

The Endocrine Society's stance on T optimization is that TTh, when initiated, should raise serum total T only up to the mid-normal range, which is approximately 426 ng/dL.[28] They also recommend that it should only be initiated when multiple unequivocal tests demonstrate low levels of serum total testosterone paired with signs and symptoms of TD. However, as recognized by the American Urological Association, there are men with total T levels greater than 300 ng/dL who exhibit conclusive and significant signs and symptoms of *hypogonadism* and have experienced symptomatic improvement with TTh. Thus, TTh aimed at raising serum total T to optimized therapeutic levels should be considered in those cases. The use of sound clinical judgment and discussing risks versus benefits with the patient is strongly encouraged.

Many studies demonstrating little or no benefit when initiating TTh provide little information about the maximum serum T levels attained in the men tested. Are the subject's serum total T levels at the low standard or mid-standard value? More research should be conducted on the impact of optimized serum T levels on symptomatic hypogonadal men.

## DISCUSSION

*T*, once touted as "the Elixir of Life," is a hormone found in both men and women. In men, most T is produced by the Leydig cells in the testicles when stimulated by the LH. T has been shown to improve bone health and density. Therapeutic levels of T also increase sexual function and libido, physical performance, strength, lean body mass, and cognitive function. However, supratherapeutic levels can cause mood swings, increased sebum production resulting in acne, elevated estradiol levels, erythrocytosis, increased incidence of male pattern baldness, and can worsen sleep apnea.

Over the last 3 decades, there has been increased interest in TTh. This trend results from increasing obesity rates, an aging population, and endocrine disruptors in our foods and environment. In addition, there has been a surge in Men's Health clinics and online direct-to-consumer Web sites, making TTh much more readily accessible. The potential risks associated with supratherapeutic levels of T have created conflicting guidelines and treatment strategies for many organizations across the globe for diagnosing and prescribing *hypogonadism*. The inconsistency of standards has led to confusion and uncertainty among prescribers. Much of the confusion lies wherein the total serum T is in the low normal range, but signs and symptoms of *hypogonadism* still exist. T optimization should be considered within this realm with close follow-up and reevaluation of signs and symptoms after initiating TTh. Clinical judgment and provider-patient discussions about risk versus benefit are necessary.

These days there are many T delivery methods to consider. Longer-acting T injections, including T cypionate and enanthate, provide more patient advantages due to convenience and effectiveness. Other delivery forms include shorter-acting formulations in the form of daily gels, creams, transdermal patches, and daily capsules. Lastly, subcutaneously inserted T pellets last up to 4 to 6 months. In men considering having children, the contraindication of T is due to its negative effect on spermatogenesis, in these men. SERMs such as enclomiphene citrate provide normalization of T levels while having positive effects on sperm counts. Although these medications have proved effective and well tolerated, SERMs are not FDA approved for treating hypogonadal men and have long been used off-label.

## SUMMARY

As more men seek to increase their T levels, more long-term random control studies are needed to gain better insight into T optimization to support the anecdotal observation commonly experienced in the practice setting. In addition, studies evaluating the risks and benefits of effective off-label treatment options such as SERMs should be considered. Lastly, an ever-growing number of women are turning to TTh. In this population, there lies tremendous opportunity for research focused on T optimization and those undergoing gender transitional care.

Video content accompanies this article at http://www.nursing.theclinics.com.

## CLINICS CARE POINTS

- The use of screening tools, like the Androgen Deficiency Men (A.D.A.M Questionnaire), is useful at the beginning of treatment and when reassessing effectiveness of treatment.
- LH and FSH are useful lab tests in determining whether someone has been primary or secondary hypogonadism and should always be included initially.

- Despite a seemingly limitless number of delivery methods for Testosterone Therapy, Injectable testosterone has remained as the most consistent and reliable.
- Because of the negative effect of testosterone on spermatogenesis, it is strongly recommended to verify full understanding by both the patient and the partner before initiating therapy.

## DISCLOSURE

The authors of this article do not have any commercial or financial conflicts of interest in addition to not having any funding sources.

## SUPPLEMENTARY DATA

Supplementary data related to this article can be found online at https://doi.org/10.1016/j.cnur.2023.07.001.

## REFERENCES

1. Brown-Séquard CE. Note on the effects produced on man by subcutaneous injections of a liquid obtained from the testicles of animals. Lancet 1889;134:105–7.
2. Tyagi V, Scordo M, Yoon RS, et al. Revisiting the role of testosterone: are we missing something? Rev Urol 2017;19(1):16.
3. Ugo-Neff G, Rizzolo D. Hypogonadism in men: updates and treatments. Jaapa 2022;35(5):28–34.
4. Lopez DS, Qiu X, Advani S, et al. Double trouble: co-occurrence of testosterone deficiency and body fatness associated with all-cause mortality in US men. Clin Endocrinol 2018;88(1):58–65.
5. Cohen J, Nassau DE, Patel P, et al. Low testosterone in adolescents & young adults. Front Endocrinol 2020;10:916.
6. Khera M, Adaikan G, Buvat J, et al. Diagnosis and treatment of testosterone deficiency: recommendations from the Fourth International Consultation for Sexual Medicine (ICSM 2015). J Sex Med 2016;13(12):1787–804.
7. Bhasin S, Lincoff AM, Basaria S, et al, TRAVERSE Study Investigators. Effects of long-term testosterone treatment on cardiovascular outcomes in men with hypogonadism: rationale and design of the TRAVERSE study. Am Heart J 2022;245:41–50.
8. Ros CTD, Ros LUD, Ros JPUD. The role of clomiphene citrate in late onset male hypogonadism. Int Braz J Urol 2022;48:850–6.
9. Bain J, Brock G, Kuzmarov I. International consulting group canadian society for the study of the aging male: response to Health Canada's position paper on testosterone treatment. J Sex Med 2007;4:558–66.
10. Salonia A, Rastrelli G, Hackett G, et al. Pediatric and adult onset hypogonadism. Nat Rev 2019;5:1–21.
11. Simpson ER, Mahendroo MS, Means GD. Aromatase cytochrome P450, the enzyme responsible for estrogen biosynthesis. Endocr Rev 1994;15:342–55.
12. Corona G, Mannucci E, Petrone L, et al. ANDROTEST: a structured interview for the screening of hypogonadism in patients with sexual dysfunction. J Sex Med 2006;3(4):706–15.
13. Morley JE, Perry HM, Kevorkian RT, et al. Comparison of screening questionnaires for the diagnosis of hypogonadism. Maturitas 2006;53(4):424–9.

14. Chen W, Liu ZY, Wang LH, et al. Are the aging male's symptoms (AMS) scale and the androgen deficiency in the aging male (ADAM) questionnaire suitable for the screening of late-onset hypogonadism in aging Chinese men? Aging Male 2013; 16(3):92–6.

15. Bernie AM, Scovell JM, Ramasamy R. Comparison of questionnaires used for screening and symptom identification in hypogonadal men. The Ageing Male 2014;17(4):195–8.

16. Crawford ED, Heidenreich A, Lawrentschuk N, et al. Androgen-targeted therapy in men with prostate cancer: evolving practice and future considerations. Prostate Cancer Prostatic Dis 2019;22(1):24–38.

17. Bhasin S, Cunningham GR, Hayes FJ, et al. Testosterone therapy in adult men with androgen deficiency syndromes: an endocrine society clinical practice guideline. J Clin Endocrinol Metab 2006;91:1995–2010.

18. Bhasin S, Brito JP, Cunningham GR, et al. Testosterone therapy in men with hypogonadism: an endocrine society clinical practice guideline. J Clin Endocrinol Metab 2018;103:1715–44.

19. Grinspon RP, Freire AV, Rey RA. Hypogondism in pediatric health: adult medicine concepts fail. Trends Endocrinol Metab 2019;30:879–90.

20. Scovell JM, Ramasamy R, Wilken N, et al. Hypogonadal symptoms in young men are associated with a serum total testosterone threshold of 400 ng/dL. BJU Int 2015;116:142–6.

21. Rastrelli G, O'Neill TW, Ahern T, et al. Symptomatic androgen deficiency develops only when both total and free testosterone decline in obese men who may have incident biochemical secondary hypogonadism: prospective results from the EMAS. Clin Endocrinol 2018;18:459–69.

22. Varimo T, Miettinen PJ, Känsäkoski J, et al. Congenital hypogonadotropic hypogonadism, functional hypogonadotropism or constitutional delay of growth and puberty? An analysis of a large patient series from a single tertiary center. Hum Reprod 2016;32:147–53.

23. Shi Z, Araujo AB, Martin S, et al. Longitudinal changes in testosterone over five years in community-dwelling men. J Clin Endocrinol Metab 2013;98:3289–97.

24. Vowles KE, McEntee ML, Julnes PS, et al. Rates of opioid misuse, abuse, and addiction in chronic pain: a systematic review and data synthesis. Pain 2015; 156:569–76.

25. Grover S, Mattoo SK, Pendharkar S, et al. Sexual dysfunction in patients with alcohol and opioid dependence. Indian J Psychol Med 2014;36:355–65.

26. Durairajanayagam D. Lifestyle causes of male infertility. Arab J Urol 2018;16: 10–20.

27. Rastrelli G, Corona G, Maggi M. Both comorbidity burden and low testosterone can explain symptoms and signs of testosterone deficiency in men consulting for sexual dysfunction. Asian J Androl 2020;22(3):265.

28. Millar AC, Lau AN, Tomlinson G, et al. Predicting low testosterone in aging men: a systematic review. CMAJ (Can Med Assoc J) 2016;188(13):E321–30.

29. Bianchi V. Metabolic syndrome, obesity paradox and testosterone level. Endocrinol Metab Syndr 2015;4(172):1–16.

30. Hackett G, Cole N, Mulay A, et al. Long-term testosterone therapy in type 2 diabetes is associated with decreasing waist circumference and improving erectile function. World J Mens Health 2020;38:68–77.

31. Gagliano-Jucá T, Basaria S. Testosterone replacement therapy and cardiovascular risk. Nat Rev Cardiol 2019;16(9):555–74.

32. Sharma R, Oni OA, Gupta K, et al. Normalization of testosterone level is associated with reduced incidence of myocardial infarction and mortality in men. Eur Heart J 2015;36(40):2706–15.

33. Corona G, Rastrelli G, Di Pasquale G, et al. Endogenous testosterone levels and cardiovascular risk: meta-analysis of observational studies. J Sex Med 2018; 15(9):1260–71.

34. FDAA Trials Tracker retrieved from. Available at: https://fdaaa.trialstracker.net/trial/NCT03518034/. Accessed March 1, 2023.

35. Rastrelli G, Corona G, Tarocchi M, et al. How to define hypogonadism? Results from a population of men consulting for sexual dysfunction. J Endocrinol Invest 2016;39:473–84.

36. Finkelstein JS, Lee H, Burnett-Bowie SA, et al. Gonadal steroids and body composition, strength, and sexual function in men. N Engl J Med 2013;369: 1011–22.

37. Kalb S, Mahan MA, Elhadi AM, et al. Pharmacophysiology of bone and spinal fusion. Spine J 2013;13:1359–69.

38. Bianchi VE. The anti-inflammatory effects of testosterone. Journal of the Endocrine Society 2019;3(1):91–107.

39. Baillargeon J, Deer RR, Kuo YF, et al. Androgen therapy and rehospitalization in older men with testosterone deficiency. Mayo Clin Proc 2016;91(No. 5):587–95. Elsevier.

40. Caliber M, Saad F. Testosterone therapy for prevention and reversal of type 2 diabetes in men with low testosterone. Curr Opin Pharmacol 2021;58:83–9.

41. Dandona P, Dhindsa S, Ghanim H, et al. Mechanisms underlying the metabolic actions of testosterone in humans: a narrative review. Diabetes Obes Metab 2021;23:18–28.

42. Skinner JW, Otzel DM, Bowser A, et al. Muscular responses to testosterone replacement vary by administration route: a systematic review and meta-analysis. J Cachexia Sarcopenia Muscle 2018;9:465–81.

43. Contreras PH, Serrano FG, Salgado AM, et al. Insulin sensitivity and testicular function in a cohort of adult males suspected of being insulin-resistant. Front Med 2018;5:190.

44. Levine H, Jørgensen N, Martino-Andrade A, et al. Temporal trends in sperm count: a systematic review and meta-regression analysis. Hum Reprod Update 2017;23:646–59.

45. Poobalan A, Aucott L. Obesity among young adults in developing countries: a systematic overview. Curr Obes Rep 2016;5:2–13.

46. Cherrier MM, Asthana S, Plymate S, et al. Testosterone supplementation improves spatial and verbal memory in healthy older men. Neurology 2001;57(1):80–8.

47. Amanatkar HR, Chibnall JT, Seo BW, et al. Impact of exogenous testosterone on mood: a systematic review and meta-analysis of randomized placebo-controlled trials. Ann Clin Psychiatry 2014;26:19–32.

48. Culig Z, Santer FR. Androgen receptor signaling in prostate cancer. Cancer Metastas- Rev. 2014;33:413–27.

49. Price L, Said K, Haaland KY. Age-associated memory impairment of logical memory and visual reproduction. J Clin Exp Neuropsychol 2004;26(4):531–8.

50. Ceder Y, Bjartell A, Culig Z, et al. The molecular evolution of castration-resistant prostate cancer. Eur Urol Focus 2016;2:506–13.

51. Parimi V, Goyal R, Poropatich K, et al. Neuroendocrine differentiation of prostate cancer: a review. Am J Clin Exp Urol 2014;2:273–85.

52. Giovannucci E, Michaud D. The role of obesity and related metabolic distur-bances in cancers of the colon, prostate, and pancreas. Gastroenterology 2007;132:2208–25.
53. Weng H, Li S, Huang JY, et al. Androgen receptor gene polymorphisms and risk of prostate cancer: a meta-analysis. Sci Rep 2017;7:40554.
54. Ide V, Vanderschueren D, Antonio L. Treatment of men with central hypogonadism: alternatives for testosterone replacement therapy. Int J Mol Sci 2020;22(1):21.
55. Rodriguez KM, Pastuszak AW, Lipshultz LI. Enclomiphene citrate for the treat-ment of secondary male hypogonadism. Expet Opin Pharmacother 2016; 17(11):1561–7.
56. Gurayah AA, Dullea A, Weber A, et al. Long vs short acting testosterone treat-ments: a look at the risks. Urology 2023;172:5–12.
57. Bhasin S, Brito JP, Cunningham GR, et al. Testosterone therapy in men with hypo-gonadism: an Endocrine Society clinical practice guideline. J Clin Endocrinol Me-tabol 2018;103(5):1715–44.

# How do the Social Determinants of Health Impact the Post-Acute Sequelae of COVID-19: A Critical Review

Joachim G. Voss, PhD, RN, ACRN[a],*, Melissa D. Pinto, PhD, RN, FAAN[b], Candace W. Burton, PhD, RN, AFN-BC, FNAP[c]

## KEYWORDS

- Post-acute sequelae of COVID-19 (PASC) • Social determinants of health • Gender
- Phenotype

## KEY POINTS

- Five studies showed a higher prevalence of PASC in females and people of older ages.
- The frequency of discrimination experiences and stress associated with those experiences increased illness severity and increased the lasting symptom count, even after adjusting for sociodemographic factors and mental/physical health conditions.
- We need community-based research that allows us to investigate PASC and its dimensions in minority populations and understand their experiences with the current health care system.

## INTRODUCTION

The COVID-19 pandemic with its significant mortality and morbidity has had far-reaching effects on the health of populations and health care systems in the United States and globally. According to the latest Center for Disease Control data from April 13th, 2023, an estimated 104,348,746 of the US population, have been infected with COVID and a total of 1,128,404 people have died because of a severe COVID infection.[1] The COVID pandemic has significantly opened our eyes to ramifications of pervasive health disparities and social determinants of health (SDoH) in the United States.[2,3] Populations such as African Americans, Native Americans, and older adults with multiple chronic disease—already rendered vulnerable by structural

---

[a] Case Western Reserve University, Frances Payne Bolton School of Nursing, Health Education Campus, 9500 Euclid Avenue, Cleveland, OH 44106, USA; [b] University of California, Irvine, Sue and Bill Gross School of Nursing, 854 Health Sciences, Irvine, CA 92697, USA; [c] University of Nevada Las Vegas School of Nursing, 4505 South Maryland Parkway, Box 453018, Las Vegas, NV 89154-3018, USA
* Corresponding author.
*E-mail address:* joachim.voss@case.edu

Nurs Clin N Am 58 (2023) 541–568
https://doi.org/10.1016/j.cnur.2023.07.004
0029-6465/23/© 2023 Elsevier Inc. All rights reserved.

factors such as poor housing, poverty, as well as inequalities based on gender identity, race, and socioeconomic status–have been further disenfranchised by lack of transportation, access to health care, and reduced public health services. These negative impacts in both social and physiologic conditions have been detrimental to the health and wellbeing of affected populations and communities.[4] Together, SDoH factors have disproportionately contributed to the high mortality and morbidity due to COVID-19 infection and given rise to the new chronic condition called long COVID or more formally referred to as post-acute syndrome of COVID-19 (PASC).[5–7] We use PASC from this point forward; it is a new chronic illness resulting from an infection with the SARS-CoV-2 virus that causes significant functional impairment and disability.[8,9]

Emerging literature has shown that PASC can impact every organ system in the human body. As such, symptom presentations vary from patient to patient, with some of the most common symptoms being fatigue, post-exertional malaise, memory and cognitive impairment, and anxiety and depression.[10]

## HISTORY

The[5,11] defines PASC as lingering symptoms that cannot be explained by any other illness or disease, that occur within 2 months of a COVID illness, and last for at least two months.[12] As of January 2023, based on new estimates between 10% and 15% of individuals who have had a history of COVID infection currently have PASC.[8–10] This means an estimated 10 to 15 million people of the US population are suffering from the long-term consequences of a COVID-19 infection. The duration of PASC symptoms is not clear at this point. Persons with lingering symptoms who contracted SARS-CoV-2 early in the pandemic have now been struggling with PASC symptoms for more than 3 years; there is no relief from symptoms or end of the illness in sight. Groff and colleagues[13] conducted a systematic review in more than 250,000 COVID survivors to investigate the short and long-term rates of PASC symptoms and found at 1 month (short-term) 54.0% experienced at least 1 PASC, at 2 to 5 months (intermediate) 55.0%, and at 6 or more months (long-term) 54.0% experienced 1 PASC symptom. PASC does not have a cure or treatment, and little is understood about the disease and many patients suffer from being taken seriously with their symptoms by their providers.[2] Given the already disproportionate effects of chronic illness on many marginalized groups, it is imperative to consider the potential impact of PASC as it may intersect with the SDoH.

## BACKGROUND
### Social Determinants of Health: Critical Perspectives

Due to the novelty of PASC as a diagnosis, it is important to contextualize the experiences of those it affects within the social environment. The application of a critical theoretic perspective offers a meaningful path to understanding how and when social determinants of health (SDoH) interact with PASC. Such a perspective is rooted in the historical foundations of critical social theory, in which a dialogic, transformation-oriented perspective allows for the interrogation of those constructs that shape the apparent realities of any social environment.[14] Such realities may be malleable or inflexible, and only through the interrogation of the constructs of which they are composed is it possible to determine which, how, and for whom this is manifest. In this review, PASC and the SDoH are examined in terms of the social constructs that are relevant to and composite in their surrounding environments, creating a critical perspective for inquiry.[15] This perspective directs attention to the interrogation of when the SDoH are considered in the context of PASC and allows for more focused interrogation of their effects on diagnosis, management, and overall patient impact.

### Post-Acute Sequelae and Trauma

The lack of clarity about PASC symptoms, prognoses, and treatments has created significant challenges in its management among both health care providers and patients. For the latter, the numerous stressors associated with help-seeking, symptom management, and overall changed health status can result in experiences that are ultimately traumatic.[16] According to the Substance Abuse and Mental Health Services Administration,[17] trauma results from "an event, series of events, or set of circumstances that is experienced by an individual as physically or emotionally harmful or life threatening and that has lasting adverse effects on the individual's functioning and physical, social, emotional, or spiritual well-being" [p 7]. While an initial COVID-19 infection could certainly meet these criteria, the ongoing nature of PASC frequently also causes alterations to both physical and cognitive capacities that in turn may force changes to relationships, professional or social activities, and family responsibilities among others.[18,19] These may also be traumatic and are likely to affect how an individual engages in sociolocation, or their interactions and self-identification within the social environment[20] in review. Changes due to the loss of employment or the loss of housing in a sociolocation after acquiring a new disease can impact a person's ability to receive support of friends and loved ones and limit access to physical resources that could assist in recovery.[20] Since the SDoH are necessarily part of the social environment, in that they are socially constructed units of influence with deterministic effects on the existence of and indeed the ontology of health, these must also be considered in relation to PASC[21]

### Social Environments and Determinants of Health

Critical examination of patients' experience of PASC in the context of the SDoH is particularly important in developing appropriate care strategies for those affected. In general, the SDoH are often construed as modifiable influences on health, but the degree to which an individual perceives and/or experiences them as modifiable can depend significantly on what resources and options are available. For example, factors such as race, age, and sexual orientation are far less modifiable than education, employment, or geographic location. Even these ostensibly modifiable factors, however, are often limited by social influences on the individual.

The array of such options is often conceptualized as social capital, indicating how much potential an individual has for change at a given point in time.[22] Where social capital is lacking, the individual's ability to influence their own sociolocation and/or mediate the effects of SDoH on their experiences is also often limited, and the impact of PASC in the social environment may be magnified. Particularly in considering the development of nursing care strategies for PASC, shared understanding of how the illness experience affects the individual across multiple life domains can enhance the patient-provider relationship and improve overall outcomes.

### Definitions

To better delineate the focus of the present review, it is thus important to specify how the SDoH are operationalized and how that provides the underpinning critical framework. All subsequent definitions of the social determinants of health are variations of the original definition by the WHO, who states that social determinants of health are the environmental factors that influence health outcomes. "They are the conditions in which people are born, grow, work, live, and age, and the wider set of forces and systems shaping the conditions of daily life. These forces and systems include economic policies and systems, development agendas, social norms, social policies and political systems."**Fig. 1**.

The Department of Health and Human Services defines them very similarly:" the conditions in the environments where people are born, live, learn, work, play, worship, and age that affect a wide range of health, functioning, and quality-of-life outcomes and risks."

While the CDC defines them as: "the nonmedical factors that influence health outcomes. They are the conditions in which people are born, grow, work, live, and age, and the wider set of forces and systems shaping the conditions of daily life."

The original WHO framework had five dimensions, with a significant number of SDoH indicators, including access and quality to education (eg, access to childcare, access to pre-school, access for low-income families, access for children with disabilities, proficiency of 8th grade reading and math levels, adolescent school attendance rates, or graduation rates), health care access and quality (eg, level of preventative services, time to be seen in an emergency department, adolescent preventative care, cancer screening for breast, lung, colorectal, and cervical cancer, and birth control services), neighborhood and the built environment (eg, reduction in crime rates among young people, broadband access, safe drinking water, exposure to unhealthy air, increase the proportion of adults that walk or bike to work), social and community context (reduction in depression and anxiety in family caregivers, increase the number of adults that vote, increase positive communication between children and their parents, increase health literacy in the population), and economic stability (reduce the proportion of people living in poverty, increase the proportion of children and adults in school, reduce household food insecurity, reduce work-related injuries), all of which impact individuals and communities directly. The CDC expanded their SDoH

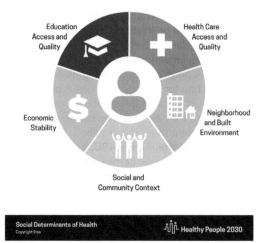

**Fig. 1.** Healthy People 2030, U.S. Department of Health and Human Services, Office of Disease Prevention and Health Promotion. Retrieved [date graphic was accessed], from https://health.gov/healthypeople/objectives-and-data/social-determinants-health

framework to six modifiable dimensions including data surveillance, evaluation and evidence building, partnership and collaboration, community engagement, infrastructure and capacity, and policy and laws. Those dimensions are seen as the drivers of equity and shape the structural and social conditions in which individuals and communities operate.

These three definitions and indicators aimed to evaluate the existing literature in terms of non-modifiable characteristics such as age, gender, race, education, pre-existing conditions, disability, as well as more structural modifiable variables such as employment, income, and community characteristics. However, in the current literature, we did not find available data on the influences of health literacy, or what role the built environment including infrastructure, public policies, partnerships, or evaluation and evidence-building played in PASC diagnosis, treatment or long-term management. Due to the existing gaps, the purpose of this article was to present the results of a systematic, critical review of PASC in the context of SDoH and to particularly consider how social structures in a world irrevocably changed by the COVID-19 pandemic may contribute to, influence, and ultimately direct outcomes among those affected by PASC.

## METHODS

We used a systematic, critical review framework to guide our work. We searched Pubmed, CINAHL, Google Scholar, and PsycInfo and used the references from current articles and conducted a hand search of the gray literature between 2019 and 2023. The search terms were quantitative and qualitative, long COVID, post-acute sequelae SARS-CoV-2 infection (PASC), social determinants of health, race, age, gender, socio-economic status, and adults and United States. Studies outside the US were excluded, as each county has very specific conditions related to SDoH, and we did not want to make direct comparisons between countries. We identified a total of 486 unique articles that were entered into an Endnote database. After careful review of titles and abstracts, and elimination of duplicates, 28 articles were read in total, and 13 articles met inclusion criteria and were eligible for our final review. Studies were included if they focused on PASC (and not just COVID infection), if they were conducted in the US, if they reported age, gender, and race as a minimum, and if they made any inferences in relation to the social determinants of health. The findings of the review are organized using the five categories: Economic stability, education access and quality, health care access, neighborhood and built environment, and social and community context.

### Quality Assessment

Once the final article selection had been made, we evaluated the overall quality of each article using the National Heart, Lung, and Blood Institute (NHLBI) Quality Assessment Tool for Observational Cohort and Cross-Sectional Studies.[23] This tool was the most appropriate because the pandemic created a specific time frame in which data collection could occur, and because most of the studies were thus necessarily observational in nature. Each article was assessed according to the 13 domains (14 items) included in the tool, and one point was awarded for each domain addressed in the article. A cutoff score of nine was deemed sufficient for inclusion in the review, and article scores ranged from nine to thirteen. See **Tables 1** and **2**.

## RESULTS

Thirteen articles met inclusion criteria. Study designs included: one qualitative, three quantitative prospective, three retrospective that used the electronic health records

**Table 1**
Article quality assessment

| 0 = no / 1 = Yes | Au, et al,[2] 2022 | Capin, et al,[8] 2022 | Estiri, et al,[9] 2021 | Frontera, et al,[24] 2022 | Goldhaber, et al,[25] 2022 | Mukherjee, et al,[26] 2022 | Pfaff, et al,[27] 2023 | Simkovich, et al,[28] 2022 | Sudre, et al,[29] 2021 | Thomason, et al,[30] 2022 | Valdes, et al,[31] 2022 | Wu, et al,[32] 2022 | Xie, et al,[33] 2022 |
|---|---|---|---|---|---|---|---|---|---|---|---|---|---|
| Question objectively stated? | 1 | 1 | 1 | 1 | 1 | 1 | 1 | 1 | 1 | 1 | 1 | 1 | 1 |
| Population specified? | 1 | 1 | 1 | 1 | 1 | 1 | 1 | 1 | 1 | 1 | 1 | 1 | 1 |
| At least 50% participation? | 1 | 1 | 1 | 1 | 1 | 1 | 1 | 1 | 1 | 1 | 1 | 1 | 1 |
| Homogenous population? In/exclusion followed? | 1 | 1 | 1 | 1 | 1 | 1 | 1 | 1 | 1 | 1 | 1 | 1 | 1 |
| Sample size justified? | 0 | 0 | 0 | 0 | 0 | 0 | 0 | 0 | 0 | 0 | 0 | 0 | 1 |
| Exposures confirmed? | 0 | 1 | 0 | 1 | 1 | 1 | 1 | 1 | 1 | 1 | 1 | 1 | 1 |
| Timeframe reasonable? | 1 | 1 | 1 | 1 | 1 | 1 | 1 | 1 | 1 | 1 | 1 | 1 | 1 |
| Different levels of exposure clear? | 0 | 0 | 0 | 0 | 0 | 0 | 0 | 0 | 0 | 0 | 0 | 0 | 1 |
| Exposure criteria clear? | 1 | 1 | 1 | 1 | 1 | 1 | 1 | 1 | 1 | 1 | 1 | 1 | 1 |
| More than one timepoint? | 0 | 1 | 1 | 1 | 1 | 1 | 1 | 1 | 1 | 1 | 1 | 1 | 1 |
| Outcomes clearly defined? | 1 | 1 | 1 | 1 | 1 | 1 | 1 | 1 | 1 | 1 | 1 | 1 | 1 |
| Blinded Experiment? | 0 | 0 | 0 | 0 | 0 | 0 | 0 | 0 | 0 | 0 | 0 | 0 | 0 |
| Loss to follow up <20%? | 1 | 1 | 1 | 1 | 1 | 1 | 1 | 1 | 1 | 1 | 1 | 1 | 1 |
| Confounders accounted? | 1 | 0 | 1 | 1 | 1 | 1 | 1 | 1 | 1 | 1 | 1 | 1 | 1 |

**Table 2**
Findings of SDOH indicators in studies of PASC patients between 2020 and 2023

| Author, Year | Design (N) | Age | Gender | Race | SDH Variable | Health Outcomes | Severity of Illness | Phenotype |
|---|---|---|---|---|---|---|---|---|
| Au, et al,[2] 2022 | Qualitative (N = 334) | Mean age = 42 | 25% male | 76% White, 4% Black, 20% other | Gender, (power, privilege, organizational structures); SES, professional dismissal | Fatigue, stress/anxiety, brain fog, cardiac, POTS, mast cell disorders | 65% infected in 2020 Participants infected in 2020 used more negative terms to describe provider interactions. | 26.8% did not continue to receive care because insurance did not cover continued treatment. |
| Capin, et al,[8] 2022 | Quantitative: physiologic + self-report instruments (N = 109) | Mean age = 53 | 51% male | 41% White, 22% Black, 31% Hispanic, 6% Other | Gender, race, | Functional performance, clinical frailty, dyspnea, disability, traumatic distress | 26% post-ICU D/C | 83% experienced new frailty or prefrailty post hospitalization and at week 18 42% still experienced frailty. |
| Estiri, et al,[9] 2021 | Quantitative: EHR review; retrospective per RT-PCR Dx using ICD-9 & 10 (N = 96,025) | Mean age = 50.7 | 36% male | 76% White, 7.5% Black, 3.5% Hispanic, 3.1% Asian | Age<65 | Alopecia, chest pain, anosmia, CFS, pneumonia, SOB, T2D, anemia, neurologic dysfunction, proteinuria | Non-hospitalized, 3–9 mo post-Dx | 33 phenotypes by age, gender, and time |

(continued on next page)

**Table 2**
*(continued)*

| Author, Year | Design (N) | Age | Gender | Race | SDH Variable | Health Outcomes | Severity of Illness | Phenotype |
|---|---|---|---|---|---|---|---|---|
| Frontera, et al,[24] 2022 | Quantitative: prospective, observational (N = 451) | Mean age T1 = 69 T2 = 65 6 and 12 mo | T1 = 65% male, T2 = 64% male | 69% White @ T1 68% White @ T2 | Age, gender, life stressors, SES, disability, social support, food insecurity | Anxiety, depression, fatigue, decreased ADL, sleep disturbance, cognitive decrease | Post-hospitalization; 34% ventilated | Old age, female sex, baseline disability, severity of COVID, life stressors worsen functional, cognitive, and neuropsychiatric outcomes |
| Goldhaber, et al,[25] 2022 | Quantitative; cross-sectional prospective cohort (N = 999) | Mean age No LC = 51.4; LC = 52.2 | No LC 56.4% LC 63.4% LC = Long CoVID | No LC = 56.8% White, 4.7% Black, 9.2% AAPI, 19.7% Other, NR 9.6% LC 50.8% White, 4.0% Black, 10.7% AAPI, 24.7% Other, NR 9.7% NR=Not reported | Age gender, race, 25 Community Characteristics known to drive health and life expectancy (Measured by Healthy Places Index (HP) domains: economic, education, health care access, housing, neighborhood clean environment, social, and transportation. | Anxiety, depressive symptoms, 16 item LC symptom specific items, self-rating of health before covid | Hospitalized 24.7%, 13% received monoclonal antibodies Included COVID + from March 1, 2020-July 1, 2021 -Includes 3 different variants (Founder, Alpha, and Delta) | 5 Symptom Clusters Emerged: Gastrointestinal, Neurocog, Musculoskeletal, Airway, and Cardiopulmonary. LC was seen 34% more in females, 4.5 times more likely after hospitalization for COVID, and were treated with monoclonal antibodies. Did not differ by race, age, or neighborhood |

| Mukherjee, et al,[26] 2022 | Self-controlled cohort design Change Health Care (United States medical claims) (N = 1.37 million) Subsample = NO LC (602,025) LC (769,085) | Mean age 55.36 | Female 59.44% | 66% White No other race was reported | Race, gender, age, income, education, and veteran status. Long-term effects of COVID-19 (determined by IC10 Codes that define LT effects) Race only was associated with "Other sepsis" alopecia area was associated with income, female gender negatively associated with sepsis and myocarditis, but positively with alopecia areata. Age was associated with most long-term consequences. | Disruption to work/school, ADL, and seeking medical care for sx. Hospital admission or treatment with monoclonal antibodies | 88% were hospitalized and 12% were in the hospital for more than 4 d | Older age was associated with LC. COVID infection was associated with subsequent malnutrition. Post-viral fatigue is associated with COVID infection. |

(continued on next page)

**Table 2**
*(continued)*

| Author, Year | Design (N) | Age | Gender | Race | SDH Variable | Health Outcomes | Severity of Illness | Phenotype |
|---|---|---|---|---|---|---|---|---|
| Simkovich et al,[28] 2022 | Cohort study of e MedStar COVID Recovery Program (N = 267) | Mean age = 47.6 | Female 76.8% | 55.4% White 32.6% Black 4.1% Asian 3% Hispanic | Age, gender, race, health insurance, employment, occupation, religion, marital status, COVID-19 management, referral to clinic, Time since COVID, symptom onset, | Participants showed reduced QOL on the PROMIS-29. Mean scores showed worse than normal QOL in all domains of the survey. Found small differences in participants <50 y of age having greater anxiety than those >50 y of age, along with greater sleep disturbance among those who are of Hispanic or other ethnic origin, and greater pain intensity and fatigue amongst females. | > 1% was ventilated 23% were hospitalized | LC patients have more social and financial impairments. |

| Pfaff, et al,[27] 2023 | EHR Retrospective Review form NC3 Data (n = 33,782) | G1 = 470,628 G2 = 795,691 G3 = 578,108 G4 = 310,304 G1<21 G2 21–45 | Female G1 = 50.7% G2 = 59.9% G3 = 54.8% G4 = 53.9% | White G1 = 52.6 G2 = 58.0 G3 = 65.2 G4 = 74.3 Black G1 = 20.3 G2 = 19.4 G3 = 17.7 G4 = 13.5 Latino G1 = 21.2 G2 = 17.2 G3 = 13.0 G4 = 6.8 | Area-level SDOH by (Zipcode): poverty, college degree, public health insurance, and unemployment, gender, age | Patients who had underlying asthma had scores that were worse than those without asthma in the domains of fatigue and ability to participate in social roles and activities. Those who were hospitalized for COVID-19 had increased impairment in physical functioning compared to those who were not hospitalized. | Using the U09.9 billing code only 9.7% were hospitalized for COVID | U09.9 patient cohort had more people below the poverty rate, had more people that were unemployed, and relied on public health insurance. People in the U09.9 cohort tended to be female, white, and non-Hispanic people. | Yes, 5 symptom clusters: neurologic, cardiopulmonary, gastrointestinal, upper respiratory, and comorbid conditions. |

*(continued on next page)*

**Table 2**
*(continued)*

| Author, Year | Design (N) | Age | Gender | Race | SDH Variable | Health Outcomes | Severity of Illness | Phenotype |
|---|---|---|---|---|---|---|---|---|
| Sudre et al,[29] 2021 | Retrospective study of COVID Symptom Study app patients (N = 4182) N = 218 from the US | Mean age G1 = 38 G2 = 50 G3 = 52 G4 = 43 G1 < 10 d G2 LC> 28 d G3 LC > 56 d G4 >10 < 28 d | % male G1 = 33 G2 = 20 G3 = 17 G4 = 28 | Not available | Location, age gender, obesity, BMI, pre-existing conditions, visit to the hospital, number of symptoms | For controls, the median duration of symptoms was 5d (3–9d), with 2.4% reporting symptoms for ≥28d. G2 was significantly associated with age, rising from 9.9% in the individuals aged 18–49 y to 21.9% in those aged ≥70 y ($P < .0005$), with an escalation in odds ratio (OR) by age decile (Fig. 1B and Supplementary Table 4). G2 disproportionately affected women (14.9%) compared with men (9.5%), | % Visit to the hospital G1 = 7 G2 = 31.5 G3 = 44 G4 = 14 | Those experiencing long COVID were consistently older, more likely to be female, and more likely to have required hospital assessment than in the group reporting symptoms for a short period of time. Those going on to experience G2 had multisystem disease from the start and needed more care. Age, sex and symptoms in the first week predicted disease duration. |

although not in
the older age
group (≥70 y).
PASC affected
all socioeconomic
groups, as
assessed using
the Index of
Multiple
Deprivation
(IMD; Extended
Data Fig. 2).
Individuals with
PASC were more
likely to have
required hospital
assessment
(see **Table 1**).
Asthma was the
only preexisting
condition
significantly
associated
with LC28
(OR = 2.14 (95%
confidence
interval (CI)
1.55–2.96)

(continued on next page)

**Table 2**
*(continued)*

| Author, Year | Design (N) | Age | Gender | Race | SDH Variable | Health Outcomes | Severity of Illness | Phenotype |
|---|---|---|---|---|---|---|---|---|
| Thomason et al,[30] 2022 | Retrospective study of early and late group of COVID patients (N = 1584) | Mean age Early = 44 Late = 45 | % male Early = 39 Late = 30.5 | %White Early = 65.5 Late = 71 % Black Early = 34.5 Late = 29 | Age, gender, marital status, education, SES risk score, Psychosocial environment Satisfaction with medical care, pre-existing medical conditions | Significant differences in early vs late infection groups were observed for composite illness severity, number of lasting symptoms, and number of lasting mood complaints after recovery. Early vs late infection groups did not differ in sociodemographic variables, including age, education, gender, marital status, race, or objective SES. | Not stated | |

| Valdes, et al,[31] 2022 | 6-mo follow-up data collected from a multi-center, prospective study of hospitalized COVID-19 patients (N = 382) | Mean age G1 = 62 G2 = 68 | % male G1 = 66 G2 = 63 | %White G1 = 59 G2 = 43 Black G1 = 7 G2 = 25 | Age, gender, race, marital status, income, education, employment, health insurance, BMI, English fluency, past medical history, baseline | Significantly different age, years of education, employment status, uninsured, race, dementia | Excluding patients with a pre-COVID history of dementia and after adjusting for univariate predictors of 6-mo t-MoCA impairment including age, Black race, years of education, pre-hospitalization employment status, primary language other than English, median household income, baseline mRS, movement disorder diagnosed during hospitalization, any neurologic event during index COVID-19 hospitalization, discharge to nursing home, |

(continued on next page)

**Table 2**
*(continued)*

| Author, Year | Design (N) | Age | Gender | Race | SDH Variable | Health Outcomes | Severity of Illness | Phenotype |
|---|---|---|---|---|---|---|---|---|
| | | | | | | | discharge to acute rehabilitation center and relevant interactions, significant, independent predictors of 6-mo t-MoCA impairment were Black race (adjusted OR 5.54, 95% CI 2.25–13.66), ≤12 y of education (adjusted OR 5.21, 95% CI 2.25–12.09), and the interaction of baseline mRS score and unemployment prior to COVID-19 hospitalization (adjusted OR 3.98, 95% CI 1.23–12.92) | |

| Wu et al,[32] 2022 | Longitudinal U.S. community population from the Understanding America Study COVID-19 Survey before, at COVID diagnosis and 12 wk after (N = 308) | Mean Age G1 = 46 G2 = 45 | %male G1 = 43 G2 = 35 | %White G1 = 61 G2 = 12 Black G1 = 62 G2 = 4 | Age, gender, race, education, smoking, current health conditions, new onset symptoms | % Obesity G1 = 42 G2 = 19 5 Headache G1 = 60 G2 = 35 Runny/stuffy nose G1 = 49 G2 = 31 Symptom count G1 = 8 G2 = 5 | People who were obese (OR = 5.44, 95% CI 2.12–13.96), and who experienced hair loss (OR = 6.94, 95% CI 1.03–46.92), headache (OR = 3.37, 95% CI 1.18–9.60), and sore throat (OR = 3.56, 95% CI 1.21–10.46) at the time of infection, had significantly higher odds of experiencing PASC | The fully adjusted logistic regression model indicates that the likelihood of experiencing PASC is not significantly associated with sociodemographic or behavioral factors including age, gender, race/ethnicity, education, current smoking status or the presence of chronic conditions. |

(continued on next page)

**Table 2**
*(continued)*

| Author, Year | Design (N) | Age | Gender | Race | SDH Variable | Health Outcomes | Severity of Illness | Phenotype |
|---|---|---|---|---|---|---|---|---|
| Xie et al,[33] 2022 | US Department of Veterans Affair COVID Cohort (181,384) | Age G1 = 62 G2 = 70 G3 = 70 | %male G1 = 88 G2 = 94 G3 = 94 | White G1 = 72 G2 = 64 G3 = 62 Black G1 = 23 G2 = 31 G3 = 32 | Age, race, health status, risk and burden of individual sequelae after 6 and 12 mo | 33 post-acute sequalae by race, gender, sex, and health status | COVID without hospitalization = 155,987 COVID without admission to ICU = 19,359 COVID with admission to ICU = 6038 | The burden of PASC increased as a function of the severity of the acute infection as proxied by the care setting and was 44.51 (43.09, 45.85), 217.08 (212.43, 222.23), and 360.16 (350.53, 369.38) per 1000 persons at 6 mo among non-hospitalized, hospitalized, and those who were admitted to intensive care during the first 30 d of infection Estimates of the burden of individual sequelae by age, race, sex, and |

baseline health status suggest a more nuanced picture in that the burden of some sequelae was more pronounced in younger adults (eg, sleep disorders, headache, mood disorders, and smell problems), Black participants (eg, new onset diabetes mellitus, chest pain, substance abuse, thromboembolism, headache, and tachycardia), and females (eg, chest pain, arrhythmia, headache, smell problems, hair loss, and skin rash)

(EHR), four retrospective that did not use the EHR, and two longitudinal cohort studies with between 6 weeks and 6 month follow-up data. Across studies, sample sizes ranged from 109 to 602,025 participants.

The demographic information on age, race/ethnicity, and sex, were captured in all studies except for Estiri, and colleagues,[9] that captured age and gender only, and constructed cohorts of age/gender for analysis using EHR data. The percentage of women in samples ranged from 0% to 75%. The mean age for men and women was 38 to 69 years of age. Racial distributions were: White 41% to 76%, Black/African American 4% to 29%, Hispanics 3% to 31%, Asians 4% to 10.7%, and others which included more than one race, or the race was not stated 6% to 24%. Other demographics included religion and marital status,[28] Body Mass Index,[29] and political identification.[2] Of the 13 studies reviewed, five studies showed a higher prevalence of PASC in females and older age which was significantly associated with higher rates of PASC.

### Economic Stability

It is well-known that individuals with greater financial resources tend to deal better with existing health problems, and economic stability is typically considered a protective factor. Across the 13 studies, economic stability was not assessed uniformly and prevented direct comparisons of findings in different groups across studies. For example, Au and colleagues (2022) assessed economic stability by employment status and total household income among a sample of predominantly white, highly educated women. This sample reported stable employment and sufficient income. Mukherjee and colleagues[26] assessed income level and reported an association between alopecia areata and two different income levels but did not specify if lower or higher income brackets experienced more alopecia areata. Pfaff and colleagues[27] included income, employment/unemployment, and identified that white women, with high levels of education, and those living in high-income neighborhoods; this group was more prone to be diagnosed with either a cardiopulmonary, neurologic, gastrointestinal, and comorbid conditions phenotype of PASC. Thomason and colleagues[30] included household income-to-needs ratio, perceived financial worries and financial satisfaction and housing stability and found no relationships between household income status and PASC. Perceived socioeconomic status was the sum of financial satisfaction, financial worries, perceived financial stability, and the score of the MacArthur ladder of perceived social standing. Valdes and colleagues[31] included median income which was determined by zip code and employment status; they found that the interaction of baseline functional status and unemployment prior to hospitalization (OR 3.98, 95%CI 1.23–12.92) was significantly associated with lower cognition as measured by the Montreal Cognitive Assessments (t-MOCA) scores.[31] Simkovich, and colleagues[28] assessed economic stability using O'Gurek', et al.[34] Social Determinants of Health Survey and found that most of their sample 72% were employed, while lacked financial resources that led to 19% not being able to afford housing and 14% could not afford food. Goldhaber, and colleagues[25,35] assessed economic stability as a component of the Health Places Index,[35] which is a weighted measure of eight components to assess health and life expectancy and is available for most neighborhoods in California. Three indicators impact economic stability are the proportion of people living above the poverty level, the proportion of people employed, and per capita income. These three indicators were compared to the other neighborhoods to assign a percentage that represents "health." Goldhaber and colleagues[25] reported no association between economic stability and PASC.

## Education Access and Quality

Goldhaber, and colleagues[25] assessed education as part of the Health Places Index and found no difference between PASC and non-PACS individuals. Pfaff, and colleagues[27] found that higher educated women were more prone to report PASC. Mukherjee,[26] Thomason, and colleagues,[30] and Wu and colleagues[32] found no relationship to education. Valdes and colleagues[31] found that lower levels of education explained higher abnormal telephone Montreal Cognitive Assessments (t-MOCA) scores.

## Health Care Access

Goldhaber, and colleagues[25] assessed health care access as a component of the Health Places Index and found no difference between individuals with PASC and those without PACS. Estiri, and colleagues[9] and Simkovich, and colleagues,[28] obtained the samples using the EHRs; therefore, the sample consisted of only persons who had access to health care. Pfaff, and colleagues,[27] and Simkovich, and colleagues,[28] captured individuals on public insurance. Simkovich and colleagues,[28] used a fairly defined inclusion criteria within the EHR, limited to individuals that engaged in health care at least twice since 2010 and the two or more visits must have been spaced at least 6 months apart. In Simkovich and colleagues,[28] all participants (N = 246) had some type or multiple forms of health insurance. Access to health insurance was not associated with PASC.

Of all the studies that met inclusion criteria, Xie, and colleagues[33] was among the most comprehensive, capturing several dimensions of health care utilization: detailed of all studies reviewed that captured several dimensions of health care utilization through the development of Area Deprivation Index. The Area Deprivation Index considered an individual's area of residence, number of outpatient encounters, number of hospital admissions, and number of outpatient prescriptions. In summary, the Area Deprivation Index captured health care use in acute and outpatient settings and in the community setting through place of residence and use of pharmacies. None of the dimensions of the Area Deprivation Index were a significant predictor in their models.

## Neighborhood and Built Environment

Few studies including neighborhood and built environment. Au[2] asked if individuals resided in urban, suburban, or rural areas. Xi, and colleagues[33] asked about residential addresses. Valdes and colleagues[31] asked about living arrangements (ie, alone, with family, nursing home, rehabilitation center or other institution) and zip code. Goldhaber and colleagues[25] was among the most comprehensive in their study of neighborhood and build environment using the Health Places Index which included neighborhood, transportation, and cleanliness of the environment. The relationships among the neighborhood, transportation, and cleanliness of the environment with PASC were not reported.

## Social and Community Context

Goldhaber, and colleagues[25] assessed social and community context as part of the Health Places Index and reported no significant relationship. Thomason, and colleagues[30] assessed two aspects of discrimination experiences frequency they occur, and stress associated with the experiences. They found that perceived discrimination increased illness severity and increased the lasting symptom count, even after adjusting for sociodemographic factors and mental/physical health conditions. COVID disease early in the pandemic was associated with a more severe illness trajectory and more frequent continuing symptoms. Finally, perceived discrimination and perceived SES increased the individual health risk. Simkovich, and colleagues[28] assessed social conditions through the Social Determinants of Health Survey and found that participants with persistent mental and physical symptoms following the initial illness reported more impairment in quality of life, socioeconomic problems, higher fatigue scores, and decreased levels of work and overall productivity.

### Additional Context from Qualitative Research

There was one qualitative study by Au, and colleagues[2] which found an overwhelming majority, 79%, of participants (individuals with PASC who engaged with health care providers) had negative interactions with providers when seeking care for PASC. "Gaslighting" was the overall summary of the participants' experience within the health care system and with health care providers.[2] Within the context of gaslighting, participants described three themes: dismissal of long COVID illness reports, prolonged diagnostic journeys, and lack of treatment options for long COVID.[2] Despite the fact that medical diagnoses are made from multiple sources of subject and objective information reported by patients in a health history, and detected by physical examination and diagnostic tests, participants report that providers used negative diagnostic findings as proof that their (the provider's) version of reality was correct and the patients were not ill or experiencing symptoms to the degree in which they were reporting.[2]

## DISCUSSION

The scant number of articles included in this review is indicative of the lack of attention that has thus far been paid to the intersection of long COVID-19 with the SDoH, even though marginalized communities have been shown to have suffered more from the pandemic than others.[36–38] There are thus several important considerations for the examination of this intersection. Firstly, given that racial and ethnic minorities experienced increased mortality during the COVID-19 pandemic, it is likely that these groups are now at greater risk of adverse impacts from other social determinants of health, such as decreased family earnings and increased family caregiving responsibilities.

The retrospective studies have focused heavily on people with access to care, on participants that carried a diagnosis of PASC, and of people with sufficient transportation so they came to their health care appointments. The prospective studies have included a majority of white, highly educated and economically stable individuals and as no surprise, they are the ones with the highest incidence in PASC (**Table 3**).

We need studies that engage equal numbers of minority participants to really understand the impact of PASC in those communities. Further, Black and Hispanic individuals are both overrepresented in "essential" non-health care service industry jobs and may be more likely to experience symptoms of PASC but are the least likely to report it.[39] This means that among these workers, employment may be unstable in the context of a chronic illness such as long COVID, and that earnings may be reduced for many. Since overall wealth has been shown to directly affect the impact of racial and ethnic disparities in health status, there may yet be far-reaching and even generational impacts of long COVID for Black, Hispanic, and Native American communities.[40,41]

Secondly, marginalized groups–those for whom the effects of the SDoH are often intensified–experience PASC in the context of intersectional, marginalized identity.

**Table 3**
Population vulnerabilities and social determinants of health domain by study

| | Population Vulnerabilities (Nonmodifiable) | Economic Stability | Education Access and Quality | Health Care Access | Neighborhood and Built Environment | Social and Community Context |
|---|---|---|---|---|---|---|
| Au et al,[2] 2022 | Age<br>Gender<br>Race/Ethnicity | X | | | X | |
| Capin et al,[8] 2022 | Age<br>Gender<br>Race/Ethnicity | | X | X | X | X |
| Estiri et al,[9] 2021 | Age<br>Gender | | | X | | |
| Frontera et al,[24] 2022 | Age<br>Gender<br>Race/Ethnicity | | X | X | X | X |
| Goldhaber et al,[25] 2022 | Age<br>Gender<br>Race/Ethnicity | X | X | X | X | X |
| Mukherjee et al,[26] 2022 | Age<br>Gender<br>Race/Ethnicity<br>Veteran Status | X | X | | | |
| Simkovich et al,[28] 2022 | Age<br>Gender<br>Race/Ethnicity<br>Marital Status | X | | X | | X |
| Pfaff et al,[27] 2023 | Age (categories)<br>Gender<br>Race/Ethnicity | X | X | X | | |

(continued on next page)

**Table 3**
*(continued)*

| | Population Vulnerabilities (Nonmodifiable) | Economic Stability | Education Access and Quality | Health Care Access | Neighborhood and Built Environment | Social and Community Context |
|---|---|---|---|---|---|---|
| Sudre et al,[29] 2021 | Age<br>Gender<br>Country of Residence (United Kingdom, Sweden, & United States) | | X | | | |
| Thomason et al,[30] 2022 | Age<br>Gender<br>Race/Ethnicity<br>Marital Status | X | X | | | X |
| Valdes et al,[31] 2022 | Age<br>Gender<br>Race/Ethnicity<br>Marital Status | X | X | X | X | |
| Wu et al,[32] 2022 | Age<br>Gender<br>Race/Ethnicity | | X | | | |
| Xie et al,[33] 2022 | Age<br>Gender<br>Race/Ethnicity | X | | X | X | |

Black and Hispanic individuals have been shown to experience more sequelae of COVID-19 illness, as well as to have less consistent access to health care in combination with increased health burdens of structural stress.[42–44] Structural stress frequently imputes an accompanying strain on both cardiovascular and inflammatory regulation via the allostatic loading process[45] both of which are systemically involved in both acute and long COVID illness.[42] In combination, the allostatic burdens of structural stress, reduced access to health care, and overall poorer outcomes of COVID-19 infection among racial and ethnic minorities are likely to intersect in ways that render affected individuals both sicker and less likely to have appropriate medical and/or economic supports.

Finally, the economic impact of long COVID on those most vulnerable to the SDoH must be considered. This impact is likely to be multifaceted, in that COVID-19 has affected employment, overall socioeconomic status (SES), and access to health care in general. Marginalized communities were more likely to experience earnings insecurity at baseline as well as reduced health care access, owing to the private insurance and health care structure in the United States, which in turn led to more severe illness from early COVID-19 infection combined with less effective or accessible treatment.[30] Among these patients, perceived discrimination and SES have been shown to increase the risk of long COVID, as does earlier and more severe infection.[30] This cyclic reinforcing of risk and impacts has the potential to eliminate those affected from the workforce as well as increase caregiving needs within families and communities. Patients with long COVID-19 are thus at risk for ongoing stress, and where health care is not effective or culturally cognizant, worsening illness and traumatic strain.[16,41]

## SUMMARY

We found that the current studies have focused heavily on populations with stable access to care, high levels of education, and come from economically better situated communities. While these data are an important first step to define specific phenotypes of a new disease, they did not reflect the communities that were most impacted by PASC. In the future, we need community-based research that allows us to investigate PASC and its dimensions in minority populations and understand their experiences with the current health care system. We learned that even well educated, financially stable, and culturally mainstream patients have experienced a high degree of gaslighting by their providers and we can only anticipate how much more difficult and traumatic the interactions are for people with PASC without those resources. More research is needed to better understand what experiences and strategies minority populations use to manage with the effects of PASC.

## CLINICS CARE POINTS

- Currently, women, older adults, people with health insurance have a higher likelihood to report symptoms related to PASC.
- Minority populations frequently experience greater financial impact of COVID, and we do not know how many experience PASC.
- Overall, 10% to 15% of people post COVID-19 infection experience at least one long term symptom for as long as 6 months.
- PASC is a complex postviral syndrome that can impact every organ-system in the body.

## DISCLOSURE

The authors report no commercial or financial conflicts of interest and any funding sources.

## REFERENCES

1. Center for Disease Control and Prevention. COVID Data Tracker. Updated July 10th, 2023. https://covid.cdc.gov/covid-data-tracker/#datatracker-home. Accessed April 14th, 2023.
2. Au L, Capotescu C, Eyal G, et al. Long covid and medical gaslighting: Dismissal, delayed diagnosis, and deferred treatment. SSM Qual Res Health 2022;2: 100167.
3. Berger Z, Altiery DE Jesus V, Assoumou SA, et al. Long COVID and Health Inequities: The Role of Primary Care. Milbank Q 2021;99(2):519–41.
4. Drake P & Rudowitz R. Tracking the Social Determinants of Health during the COVID-19 pandemic. KFF. April 21, 2021. https://www.kff.org/coronavirus-covid-19/issue-brief/tracking-social-determinants-of-health-during-the-covid-19-pandemic. Accessed April, 28, 2023.
5. World Health Organization. A clinical case definition of post-COVID-19 condition by a Delphi consensus, 2021. https://www.who.int/publications/i/item/WHO-2019-nCoV-Post_COVID-19_condition-Clinical_case_definition-2021.1. Accessed May 10th, 2023.
6. U.S. Department of Health and Human Services, Office of Disease Prevention and Health Promotion. Healthy People 2030. 2021. https://health.gov/healthypeople/objectives-and-data/social-determinants-health. Accessed April 13th, 2023.
7. Center for Disease Control. NCHHSTP Social Determinants of Health, 2022. https://www.cdc.gov/nchhstp/socialdeterminants/index.html#:~:text=Social%20determinants%20of%20health%20(SDOH,the%20conditions%20of%20daily%20life. Accessed April 13, 2023.
8. Capin JJ, Wilson MP, Hare K, et al. Prospective telehealth analysis of functional performance, frailty, quality of life, and mental health after COVID-19 hospitalization. BMC Geriatr 2022;22(1):251.
9. Estiri H, Strasser ZH, Brat GA, et al. Evolving phenotypes of non-hospitalized patients that indicate long COVID. BMC Med 2021;19(1):249.
10. Nalbandian A, Desai AD, Wan EY. Post-COVID-19 Condition. Annu Rev Med 2023;74:55–64.
11. World Health Organization. COVID-19 and the Social Determinants of Health and Health Equity: evidence brief. December 6, 2021. https://www.who.int/publications/i/item/9789240038387. Accessed, April 2, 2023.
12. WHO REFERENCE NUMBER: WHO/2019-nCoV/Post_COVID-19_condition/Clinical_case_definition/2021.1
13. Groff D, Sun A, Ssentongo AE, et al. Short-term and Long-term Rates of Post acute Sequelae of SARS-CoV-2 Infection: A Systematic Review. JAMA Netw Open 2021;4(10):e2128568.
14. Collins PH. Intersectionality as critical social theory. Duke University Press; 2019.
15. Gannon S, Davies B. Postmodern, Post-Structural, and Critical Theories. In: Hesse-Biber SN, editor. The Handbook of feminist research: theory and praxis. 2nd edition. SAGE; 2012. p. 65–91.

16. Burton CW, Downs CA, Hughes T, et al. A novel conceptual model of trauma-informed care for patients with post-acute sequelae of SARS-CoV-2 illness (PASC). J Adv Nurs 2022;78(11):3618–28.
17. Substance Abuse and Mental Health Services Administration. SAMHSA's Concept of Trauma and Guidance for a Trauma-Informed Approach. July 2014, https://store.samhsa.gov/system/files/sma14-4884.pdf. Accessed May 25, 2023.
18. Davis HE, Assaf GS, McCorkell L, et al. Characterizing long COVID in an international cohort: 7 months of symptoms and their impact. EClinicalMedicine 2021; 38:101019.
19. Ziauddeen N, Gurdasani D, O'Hara ME, et al. Characteristics and impact of Long Covid: Findings from an online survey. PLoS One 2022;17(3):e0264331.
20. Burton CW, Downs CA, Hughes T, et al. A novel conceptual model of trauma-informed care for patients with post-acute sequelae of SARS-CoV-2 illness (PASC). J Adv Nurs 2022;78(11):3618–28.
21. Braveman P, Gottlieb L. The social determinants of health: it's time to consider the causes of the causes. Public Health Rep 2014;129(Suppl 2):19–31.
22. Moore S, Kawachi I. Twenty years of social capital and health research: a glossary. J Epidemiol Community Health 2017;71(5):513–7.
23. National Heart, Lung, and Blood Institute. Study Quality Assessment Tools. July 2021. https://www.nhlbi.nih.gov/health-topics/study-quality-assessment-tools. Accessed, April 13, 2023.
24. Frontera JA, Sabadia S, Yang D, et al. Life stressors significantly impact long-term outcomes and post-acute symptoms 12-months after COVID-19 hospitalization. J Neurol Sci 2022;443:120487.
25. Goldhaber NH, Kohn JN, Ogan WS, et al. Deep Dive into the Long Haul: Analysis of Symptom Clusters and Risk Factors for Post-Acute Sequelae of COVID-19 to Inform Clinical Care. Int J Environ Res Public Health 2022;19(24):16841.
26. Mukherjee S, Kshirsagar M, Becker N, et al. Identifying long-term effects of SARS-CoV-2 and their association with social determinants of health in a cohort of over one million COVID-19 survivors. BMC Publ Health 2022;22(1):2394.
27. Pfaff ER, Madlock-Brown C, Baratta JM, et al. Coding long COVID: characterizing a new disease through an ICD-10 lens. BMC Med 2023;21(1):58.
28. Simkovich SM, Ahmed N, Chou J, et al. Health, social, and economic characteristics of patients enrolled in a COVID-19 recovery program. PLoS One 2022; 17(11):e0278154.
29. Sudre CH, Murray B, Varsavsky T, et al. Attributes and predictors of long COVID [published correction appears in Nat Med. 2021 Jun;27(6):1116]. Nat Med 2021; 27(4):626–31.
30. Thomason ME, Hendrix CL, Werchan D, et al. Perceived discrimination as a modifier of health, disease, and medicine: empirical data from the COVID-19 pandemic. Transl Psychiatry 2022;12(1):284.
31. Valdes E, Fuchs B, Morrison C, et al. Demographic and social determinants of cognitive dysfunction following hospitalization for COVID-19. J Neurol Sci 2022; 438:120146.
32. Wu Q, Ailshire JA, Crimmins EM. Long COVID and symptom trajectory in a representative sample of Americans in the first year of the pandemic. Sci Rep 2022; 12(1):11647.
33. Xie Y, Bowe B, Al-Aly Z. Burdens of post-acute sequelae of COVID-19 by severity of acute infection, demographics and health status. Nat Commun 2021;12(1): 6571.

34. O'Gurek DT, Henke C. A Practical Approach to Screening for Social Determinants of Health. Fam Pract Manag 2018;25(3):7–12.
35. Public Health Alliance Southern California. California Healthy Place Index. 2022. https://www.healthyplacesindex.org/. Accessed, May 10, 2023.
36. Caraballo C, Massey DS, Ndumele CD, et al. Excess Mortality and Years of Potential Life Lost Among the Black Population in the US, 1999-2020. JAMA 2023;329(19):1662–70.
37. Andrasfay T, Goldman N. Reductions in US life expectancy during the COVID-19 pandemic by race and ethnicity: Is 2021 a repetition of 2020? PLoS One 2022; 17(8):e0272973.
38. Goldman N, Andrasfay T. Life expectancy loss among Native Americans during the COVID-19 pandemic. Demogr Res 2022;47:233–46.
39. Jacobs MM, Evans E, Ellis C. Racial, ethnic, and sex disparities in the incidence and cognitive symptomology of long COVID-19. J Natl Med Assoc 2023;115(2): 233–43.
40. Sun S, Lee H, Hudson DL. Racial/ethnic differences in the relationship between wealth and health across young adulthood. SSM Popul Health 2022;21:101313.
41. DeWilde C, Burton CW. Cultural Distress: An Emerging Paradigm. J Transcult Nurs 2017;28(4):334–41.
42. Khullar D, Zhang Y, Zang C, et al. Racial/Ethnic Disparities in Post-acute Sequelae of SARS-CoV-2 Infection in New York: an EHR-Based Cohort Study from the RECOVER Program. J Gen Intern Med 2023;38(5):1127–36.
43. Burton CW, Gilpin CE, Draughon Moret J. Structural violence: A concept analysis to inform nursing science and practice. Nurs Forum 2021;56(2):382–8.
44. Burton CW, Gilpin CE, & Draughon Moret J. Structural violence: A concept analysis to inform nursing science and practice. Nursing Forum, 1-7. 2022. Available at: https://onlinelibrary.wiley.com/doi/abs/10.1111/nuf.12535. Accessed May 30, 2023.
45. Berkowitz RL, Gao X, Michaels EK, et al. Structurally vulnerable neighborhood environments and racial/ethnic COVID-19 inequities. Cities Health 2021;5(Suppl 1):S59–62.

# Men's Health as a Telehealth Strategy

Michael Ward, MSN, APRN, AGACNP-BC

## KEYWORDS

- Men's health • Telehealth • Telemedicine • Sexual medicine • Direct-to consumer

## KEY POINTS

- The emerging field of Telehealth is experiencing exponential growth in many medical specialties because of renewed interest catalyzed by the coronavirus disease 2019 pandemic.
- Men's Health is a relatively newer subspecialty, which focuses on health issues related to, but not limited to hypogonadism, erectile dysfunction, Peyronie disease, male infertility, and benign prostatic hyperplasia.
- Telehealth ameliorates apprehension in men from seeking health-care services by removing many of the perceived barriers to treatment in walk-in clinics.
- Technology has allowed Telehealth services to be increasingly accessible and affordable, with many telehealth platforms now being created for tablets and smartphones.
- Direct to consumer online Men's Health platforms are now becoming increasingly prevalent across the United States.

## INTRODUCTION

In 2020, the onslaught of the coronavirus disease 2019 (COVID-19) pandemic, both at home and abroad, resulted in unprecedented and debilitating turmoil on the health-care industry, its institutions, and those who work within. Conversely, during the same time, many employed within certain sectors of health care were found out of work or furloughed.[1,2]

Because many nonemergent medical services were closed, many medical practices, as well as patients, were forced to embrace a newer technology. The doors of the emerging field of telehealth medicine or "telemedicine" were flung wide open as COVID-19 closed the doors of many medical practices across the world.[3] As health practitioners and patients alike were mostly reluctant to assimilate to this "new" technological environment, many discovered this approach to provide convenience, comfort, and cost-effective care during a time it was most needed.[4]

Critical Care Nurse Practitioner, Cardiovascular ICU, Medical ICU, Texas Health Huguley Hospital, 924 Yarwood Way, Burleson, TX 76028, USA
E-mail address: Brandonw.rn@gmail.com

Nurs Clin N Am 58 (2023) 569–580
https://doi.org/10.1016/j.cnur.2023.07.002
0029-6465/23/© 2023 Elsevier Inc. All rights reserved.
nursing.theclinics.com

As the world has now returned to near normalcy and health-care workers have returned to their positions, many patients and providers have continued to embrace telehealth medicine.[5] Platforms providing only telehealth services have begun springing up online and all across the United States.[6] Additionally, an increasing number of medical practices now provide both in-office visits and telehealth services for encounters, which do not require a hands-on physical examination. One of the specialties who have seen tremendous growth with the utilization of Telehealth services is one of the newer subspecialties within health care, men's health. The purpose of this article is to discuss men's health and examine the advantages and disadvantages of men's health as a telehealth strategy.

## MEN'S HEALTH

Despite the many known gender differences in respect to health outcomes, *Men's Health* is a relatively newer term within Medicine. Men's health, sometimes referred to as andrology, is often considered a subset of urology and was not a hot topic until sildenafil was first identified to improve erectile dysfunction (ED) in 1999. It was subsequent emerging data that ED in younger men could potentially indicate an increased risk of future cardiac events that the discussion turned toward gender-related health disparities (**Fig. 1**).[7]

Historically, it has been shown that men and women are disproportionately proactive in their involvement in health maintenance and overall health in general. Men far less frequently visit their primary care providers or seek out medical assistance at all, despite higher risks for heart disease, cancer, diabetes, suicide, alcoholic liver disease, increased risk taking behaviors, and other morbidities.[8] In addition, it has been shown that men live approximately 5 years fewer than women do on average.[9]

This reluctance has been demonstrated to be multifactorial in nature but is primarily attributed to one of the major social determinants of health, male gender norms, more specifically, ideas of traditional masculinity.[10] The medical literature is replete with examples that illustrate this point. In one recent study by Novak and colleagues, male participants aged 21 to 82 years were asked in 5 semistructured focus groups the question, "Some people say that men avoid going to the doctors or reporting their illness. Is this true for you? Why or why not?" Some of the responses included "men don't go to the doctor," "men are supposed to push through the pain," and "if it's not broken, don't fix it."[11]

The outcome of the study determined that the notion of societal male norms plays a large role in this behavior.[11] Other reasons for avoidance of health care include embarrassment, fear of dismissiveness by their provider, cost, and inconvenience.[12]

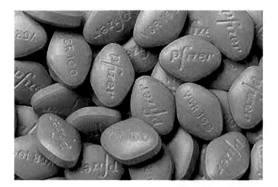

**Fig. 1.** Viagra.

This avoidance seems to be exacerbated in the face of many common male issues surrounding sexual dysfunction: ED, hypogonadism, male infertility, Peyronie disease, and lower urinary tract symptoms (LUTS)—or in whole, men's health.

## ERECTILE DYSFUNCTION

ED is characterized as an inability to maintain or sustain an erection for sexual performance and is quite common among middle-aged men. According to Rodler and colleagues, the diagnosis of ED is commonly missed in patient examinations due to several reasons. Some of which include lack of consideration by the provider, embarrassment by both the patient and provider and false patient beliefs.[13] Interestingly, approximately 50% of men between the ages of 40 and 70 years are impacted and the presence of ED can be a potential implication of underlying cardiac disease, metabolic syndrome, and hypogonadism.[12] Despite this, it is still stigmatized among men and considered a topic of avoidance.

## HYPOGONADISM

Hypogonadism in men is defined by the Endocrine Society as a clinical syndrome that results from failure of the testes to produce physiological levels of testosterone due to the disruption of one or more levels of the hypothalamic-pituitary-testicular axis.[14] It can be classified as primary or secondary and can result from many causes. Known contributing factors include obesity, diabetes, environmental endocrine disruptors, and aging. Symptoms may include low libido, fatigue, loss of lean muscle mass, sexual dysfunction, and depression.[15] It is estimated that 2 to 4 million men in the United States have hypogonadism. One in 10 men aged older than 60 years and 1 in 3 men with diabetes are affected.[16] Although, this number may be higher.

## MALE INFERTILITY

Infertility is classified as the inability to conceive after 1 full year of unprotected intercourse. It is estimated that 186 million people globally are affected by infertility and men contribute to about half of all cases.[17] Male infertility is based on semen analysis and causes include hormonal disorders, physical, psychological, sexual, and chromosomal problems.[18] Despite many known reasons for male infertility, researchers are unable to determine the underlying cause in approximately 70% of those cases.[18]

## PEYRONIE DISEASE

Peyronie disease is a fibrosing condition, which causes scarring and contractures within the tunica albuginea of the penis.[19] This results in sometimes severe and painful curvature of the penis and can result in emotional and psychological stress on both the male and partner.[20] Treatment depends on the severity of the disease. However, without treatment, the problem can remain stable or likely worsen over time.

## LOWER URINARY TRACT SYMPTOMS

Benign prostatic hyperplasia (BPH) is the leading cause of LUTS including bladder outlet obstruction and is closely linked to ED. It has been quipped that it is not a matter of *if* a man will have BPH but a matter of *when*. According to the most recent data, BPH affects 50% of men aged from 50 to 59 years and 90% of men aged older than 80 years.[21]

As we reexamine the number of men affected by sexual dysfunction, it is conceivable that most men will experience some sort of sexual dysfunction within their lifetime.

However, Laumann and colleagues[22] demonstrated in a recent study that less than 25% of men with sexual dysfunction actually sought medical care at all. As the topic of Men's Health has become more mainstream, due in part by many national and international campaigns to bring about men's health awareness, many men have begun turning to a newer medical option: enter the men's health clinic.

## MEN'S HEALTH CLINICS

Traditionally, men have not had access to gender-specific specialists or health-care initiatives aimed solely at improving the health of men. In 2016, the American Urological Association (AUA) census revealed that approximately 62% of counties in the United States have no urologists at all.[23] Conversely, gynecologists have been treating women for some time now. The oldest record we have detailing gynecological care was composed in 1800 BC and is called the Kahun Gynecological Papyrus and is from the 12th Egyptian Dynasty. Despite health care reluctance by many men, it has also been contested that this lack of specialized care has contributed to premature male mortality and higher risks for the aforementioned morbidities than in women **(Fig. 2)**.[24]

Today, however, it is now not uncommon in any metropolitan area to drive past one or more men's health clinics on a daily commute. During the past 2 decades, the number of men's health clinics has skyrocketed across the United States. The majority of these clinics offer therapies that are geared toward improving sexual health in men, mostly hypogonadism, infertility, and ED. Because men's health encompasses more than solely sexual dysfunction, additional options are now increasingly becoming available.

Just during the last decade, multidisciplinary academic centers have begun embracing men's health, providing comprehensive medical care in which, in addition to urologic and sexual health issues, they offer care for mental health, addiction health, cardiology, dermatology, and even hair loss.[25] Unfortunately, in more rural areas of the country, there is a paucity of these men's health clinics and multidisciplinary centers. This is one of the many reasons telehealth has begun gaining popularity within the realm of men's health.

## TELEHEALTH

Although it seems the advent of telehealth or *telemedicine*, often used interchangeably, is a new technology, it only seems so after it was thrust back into the spotlight because of the severe acute respiratory syndrome coronavirus 2 (SARS-Co-V2) global pandemic in March of 2020. The idea of telehealth, however, has been around for nearly 145 years! As early as 1879, the notion of Telehealth was mentioned by the

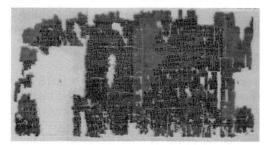

**Fig. 2.** Kahun gynecological papyrus.

*Lancet* as a means to use the telephone to reduce the number of office visits by patients.[26] The front cover of *Science and Invention* magazine in 1925 interestingly showed a depiction of a physician with ear buds performing a physical examination on a patient by video from his desk. In April of 1968, the Logan International Airport Massachusetts General Hospital Medical Station launched a "Telediagnosis" program that actually did just that (**Figs. 3** and **4**).[27]

There have been many other examples where telehealth strategies have been used over that time. Because of the SARS-CoV-2 outbreak in early 2020, an unprecedented and rapid transition to telehealth and telemedicine by most medical practices and hospitals globally was made in an attempt to reduce and prevent the spread of the virus. Medical specialties such as dermatology, psychology, radiology, and even dentistry have all now used telehealth as a platform to diagnose and treat patients.[27]

Before the COVID-19 pandemic, the use of telehealth by men's health physicians was minimal. According to a 2019 institutional study, only 14% of surveyed urologists implemented telehealth within their practice. About 70% of these urologists cited low reimbursements to be the number one causative factor.[28] Because medical practices were quickly forced to adopt the use of telemedicine in 2020, legislation also made swift moves to expand coverage for telemedicine health-care services.[29]

Since that time, a large increase in the use of telehealth among urologists has occurred. A 2020 cross-sectional analysis revealed that the use of telehealth among urologists during the COVID-19 pandemic tripled globally.[30] About 81% of the same urologists found that the use of telemedicine to be overall useful within their practices and claimed they intended on continuing its use indefinitely. Rabinowitz and colleagues[31] conducted a study to examine the importance of telehealth visits for the treatment of men's health patients at a major academic center and concluded that telemedicine was indeed compatible with the field of men's health.

## ADVANTAGES OF TELEHEALTH

Increasing costs of health care, physician shortages, and lack of immediate access in rural communities are only a few of the many issues for which solutions are offered

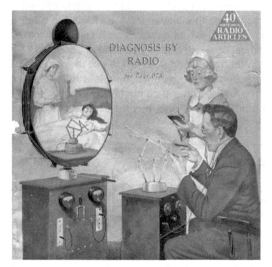

**Fig. 3.** 'Science and Invention' Magazine Cover of February 1925 issue. *Retrieved from* https://worldradiohistory.com/Archive-Electrical-Experimenter/SI-1925-02.pdf.

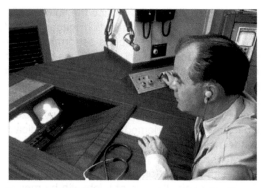

**Fig. 4.** Massachusetts general hospital archives and special collections.

through telehealth. It is clear that the implementation of telehealth has its advantages. Dorsey and colleagues[32] expounds on this as they discuss the 5C's of telemedicine: *care*, *convenience*, *comfort*, *confidentiality*, and *contagion*.

Care, meaning *access to care*. As mentioned, because of the severe lack of men's health specialists in many communities in the United States, it is sometimes difficult for men to visit a men's health provider. The use of telehealth removes any geographical limitations or barriers that arise from a lack of local care.

*Convenience* is exemplified by the ability to receive care while remaining at home or wherever you may be, as long as you have access to the Internet. During a normal work week, many men have to take off work to visit their provider. With telemedicine, it can be as convenient as closing the office door and seeing your provider over the phone or computer, and then get right back to work.

Many men are uncomfortable talking to a medical provider about their health problems, especially when it involves sexual dysfunction. This is associated with the perceived stigma of men seeking medical care. With telehealth, men can visit their provider in the *comfort* of their own home in private. This particular advantage has led to the explosive growth seen in web-based men's telehealth platforms.

Similar to comfort, many men prefer the *confidentiality* offered by telemedicine. In person visits at a men's health clinic announces to all the other men in the waiting room "I have some type of sexual dysfunction." Telemedicine offers a safe haven for men to seek medical care without many of those concerns.

Finally, *contagion*. When attending an in-office visit to your medical provider, there is always a risk of contracting an illness from someone either in the medical office or from someone with whom you may come in contact. The use of telemedicine eliminates the risk of contracting other illnesses one may be exposed to during an in-person visit (**Box 1**).

---

**Box 1**
**Dorsey's 5 C's of telemedicine**

(*Adapted from* Dorsey ER, Okun MS, Bloem BR. Care, Convenience, Comfort, Confidentiality, and Contagion: The 5 C's that Will Shape the Future of Telemedicine. Journal of Parkinson's Disease. 2020;10(3):893-897. https://doi.org/10.3233/JPD-202109.)

    Care
    Convenience
    Comfort
    Confidentiality
    Contagion

## DISADVANTAGES

Although there are many advantages with the use of telehealth, it also brings with it some disadvantages. These include technological barriers among older patients, minority patients, and non–English-speaking patients. Additionally, in some rural communities, bandwidth speeds have been shown to be problematic. With telemedicine, the lack of an actual hands-on physical examination is a significant barrier, arguably the most concerning. However, with men's health, many of these issues men face can still be thoroughly treated without a hands-on physical examination.[33] As technology continues to advance over time and people become more accustomed to the use of telehealth, the feasibility of treating patients remotely will also continue to improve.

## REIMBURSEMENT/COST

Yet, concerns remain among health-care providers involving regulatory barriers and lack of significant reimbursements.[34] The Public Health Emergency (PHE) declaration lifted restrictions for many of the constraints found within the use of telehealth. These restrictions included the prescribing of controlled substances without an in-person visit and reimbursement for telehealth services for Medicaid and Medicare patients. Until recently, there has been little clarity about what the new norm will be when the PHE declaration will be removed and what that will mean for the many patients and providers that have adjusted to the use of telehealth services.

As of November 2021, Centers for Medicare and Medicaid Services (CMS) have released the final version of the Calendar Year 2023 Medicare Physician Fee Schedule and an accompanying fact sheet. This document has included new reimbursement codes for the use of telehealth technology. Also discussed within that document is which services will be covered by the program and what will happen immediately following the end of the PHE. See full document at https://public-inspection.federalregister.gov/2022-23873.pdf.

Photo: Final CY 2023 Physician Fee Schedule Fact Sheet.

## DIRECT TO CONSUMERS MEN'S HEALTH PLATFORMS

Before the COVID-19 pandemic, direct to consumer (DTC) men's health platforms were increasing. From 2017 to 2019, there was a notable increase of 1500% in visitors to these online platforms, with more than 11 million visits in just the last quarter of 2019.[12] Most of these platforms such as HIMS, Hone Health, and MaleExcel provide men's health services in the form of fertility treatment, ED medications, male pattern balding medications, and testosterone replacement therapies.

Much controversy surrounds these online clinics because of the concern with the lack of guideline-concordant care.[35] Many who oppose these online platforms think there is a lack of transparency regarding the negative impact these medications can potentially have on patients. Additional concerns involve lack of routine follow-ups and off-label misuse of these therapies. Nonetheless, the growth of these platforms continues. One line of thought is that they fulfill a need by patients who live in communities that lack available urological services. Additionally, they provide convenience and affordability. Demaerschalk and colleagues[36] demonstrated that the average cost savings with each telemedicine visit was approximately US$888 when all the costs associated with the visit (travel, meals, accommodations, and missed work) were considered.

Testosterone is a scheduled III controlled medication. For this reason, concerns are mounting by both patients and prescribers whether or not the new laws will influence care delivery through these DTC web-based men's health platforms that offer testosterone therapies when they take effect. Up until now, there has been little governmental clarity in this area. Interestingly, the AUA does not require either a physical examination or digital rectal examination for prostate screening as a requirement for the initiation of testosterone replacement therapy.[37,38] Therefore, web-based men's health platforms that provide testosterone therapy are a feasible option as for now.

## FUTURE OF MEN'S TELEHEALTH

As the landscape of telehealth is evolving, so too is the landscape of men's health. As more and more men turn to men's health clinics for their care, it will require a multidisciplinary approach by providers who are comfortable with various men's health issues. At this time, there are 15 men's health fellowships around the nation, including programs at UCLA, Northwestern, and Baylor University.[7] This number is expected to grow in time. As more of these programs develop, the result will be more qualified men's health providers to meet the increasing demand for patients seeking men's health services.

Additionally, with advancements in telehealth software and hardware, the feasibility to which telehealth is implemented is continually improving. These days it is as easy for a patient to connect to a provider as it is turning on their phone. With a simple touch of a button on a smartphone or tablet, a patient can be connected in seconds. Apps such as Doxy.me, WhatsApp, and Skype are available for download on all platforms. This ease of use is also being observed by men's health providers. Medical software developers such as EpicCare, Cerner Ambulatory, and Optimantra now provide fully integrated Health Insurance Portability and Accountability Act (HIPAA)compliant telehealth software within the electronic medical record.

Telehealth examination medical devices, also known as telehealth *peripherals*, provide the medical provider the ability to physically assess patients who may visit a nurse-staffed satellite office in a rural community. These devices include electronic stethoscopes, tele-opthalmoscopes, video-otoscopes, electronic dermatoscopes, and digital endoscopes.[39]

## CLINICAL DISCUSSION/IMPLICATIONS

This article sought to discuss men's health and examine the advantages and disadvantages of men's health as a telehealth strategy. There has been considerable scholarship demonstrating that biological males are sociologically predisposed to increased health risks and have higher rates of morbidity and mortality than their biological female counterparts. This has been identified largely because of decreased health-seeking behavior related to traditional masculine norms, the stigmatization of men seeking medical care, and the stigma associated with male sexual dysfunction.[6,7,11–13,31,35] Other reasons of avoidance included the lack of men's health services regionally, inconvenience, and cost.

Historically, urologists and other men's health providers have been reluctant to integrate telehealth into their medical practices. Barriers to implementation included a lack of technological literacy, concerns for the provision of inadequate treatment (ie, lack of hands-on physical examinations), and financial reimbursements.[30,40] The latter expressed as the most concerning, statistically. It was not until the COVID-19 pandemic that the number of men's health providers' use of telehealth surged. The percentage of urologists surveyed by Dubin and colleagues[30] showed an increase of nearly 200% in their adoption of telehealth during the pandemic with approximately 81% of those interested in its continued use indefinitely. In combination with the notable increase and year over year growth in online men's health DTC websites, such as HIMS, Hone Health, and MaleExcel, we are observing a paradigm shift in men's health care in real time.

Because of the complexity associated with men's health, some academic health-care institutions are taking a multidisciplinary approach to men's health, offering telehealth services and treatment not only in sexual dysfunction but also in physical performance and psychological issues.[7] Institutions, such as Baylor University, UCLA, and Northwestern, are bringing more men's health specialists to the front because these and others are focusing their efforts on creating men's health Fellowships to combat the dearth of providers within the specialty.

Because the PHE declaration is soon coming to an end, there has been little legislative clarity and guidance on the implementation of telehealth services. This concern is felt by both patients and providers. However, the CMS' recent release of the 2023 Calendar Year Physician Fee Schedule, which includes reimbursement codes specifically targeted at telehealth integration, has further solidified the perceived need for telehealth services.

## LIMITATIONS/FUTURE CONSIDERATIONS

The implementation of telemedicine within the realm of men's health has proven to be a useful tool to overcome many barriers that have historically prevented men from seeking medical care. Much of the available literature on this topic is relatively recent because the largest driver to transition from a clinic-based model to a telehealth-integrated model was a result of the recent COVID-19 pandemic. Therein lies opportunity for future research. Studies should be aimed at how the increasing use of telehealth among men is influencing health outcomes, particularly those key health issues where men surpass women in health risks, morbidity, and mortality.

Although during the past 3 years there has been a dramatic increase in the number of men using telehealth and web-based men's health clinics, according to the CDC, women still outpace men in their use of telehealth, 43% vs 31.7%, respectively.[8] Additionally, increased use of telehealth has shown to correspond with education level; household family income[8]; and inversely correlate with community size, older age, and non-English speakers.[29,31]

Unfortunately, within rural communities, lack of technical and digital literacy, as well as the lack of availability in high-speed Internet services, are obstacles to telehealth use. Future interventions, in order to promote health equity, may wish to include multilingual community led workshops on the use of video conferencing software or medical practice, web-based, video training via social media (Facebook Groups, YouTube, Vimeo, Twitter) in order to facilitate increased understanding and comfortability of these platforms. Exploration of community-based organizations across the United States, which offer low-cost high-speed Internet services with campaigns focused on bringing awareness of these options into rural communities, would also be of benefit.

## SUMMARY

Although telehealth seems to be an emerging technological marvel, it has been used in some way for many years now. Moreover, although the COVID-19 pandemic wreaked horrific and tragic havoc around the world, it brought with it a new era of patient-centered care that forced many reluctant providers to adopt its use. As a result, we are experiencing a time now where more and more men are choosing to seek medical care and treatment in an environment that provides care, convenience, comfort, and confidentiality, whereas ameliorating the risk of contracting additional illness.

Although legislation has not yet provided all the answers to the many questions that remain, it is clear that telehealth is here to stay. With newer technologies at our fingertips and on the horizon and an increased number of qualified men's health specialists coming to the fore, men's telehealth will increasingly continue to provide a viable option for men seeking care and treatment.

## CLINICS CARE POINTS

- It is paramount that, as health-care providers, we must explore methods and approaches that facilitate the destigmatization of male health-seeking behaviors because of traditional masculinity.
- Embracing and implementing telehealth services within the realm of Men's Health can potentially foster increased male participation and adherence to prescribed therapies and treatments.
- The creation of additional Men's Health fellowships in academic institutions around the United States would aid in the provision of more qualified providers of Men's Health services.

## REFERENCES

1. Oster, PhD, MPH NV, Skillman, MS SM, Frogner, PhD BK. COVID-19's Effect on the Employment Status of Health Care Workers. FamilyMedicine.uw.edu. family medicine.uw.edu/chws/wp-content/uploads/sites/5/2021/05/Health_Employ_Status_PB_May_26_2021.pdf. Published May 2021. Accessed February 28, 2023.
2. Rogowski JA. Unanticipated Consequences: Lack of Essential and Nonessential Patient Care, Furloughs of Health Care Providers, and Institutional Financial Losses. Nurses and COVID-19: Ethical Considerations in Pandemic Care 2022;63–76. https://doi.org/10.1007/978-3-030-82113-5_6.
3. Mann DM, Chen J, Chunara R, et al. COVID-19 transforms health care through telemedicine: Evidence from the field. J Am Med Inform Assoc 2020;27(7): 1132–5.
4. 2021 Telehealth Survey Report | AMA. Available at: www.ama-assn.org/system/files/telehealth-survey-report.pdf. Accessed February 28, 2023.
5. Barberio JA, Jenkins ML. Transitioning to telehealth: today's guidelines for future sustainability. J Nurse Pract 2021. https://doi.org/10.1016/j.nurpra.2021.04.001.
6. Balasubramanian A, Yu J, Srivatsav A, et al. A review of the evolving landscape between the consumer Internet and men's health. Transl Androl Urol 2020; 9(Suppl 2):S123–34.
7. Houman JJ, Eleswarapu SV, Mills JN. Current and future trends in men's health clinics. Transl Androl Urol 2020;9(Suppl 2):S116–22.
8. Acciai F, Firebaugh G. Why did life expectancy decline in the United States in 2015? A gender-specific analysis. Soc Sci Med 2017;190:174–80.
9. Arias E, Xu J, Kochanek KD. United states life tables, 2016. Natl Vital Stat Rep 2019;68(4):1–66. Available at: https://pubmed.ncbi.nlm.nih.gov/31112121/. Accessed March 1, 2023.
10. Fleming PJ, Agnew-Brune C. Current trends in the study of gender norms and health behaviors. Current Opinion in Psychology 2015;5:72–7.

11. Novak JR, Peak T, Gast J, et al. Associations between masculine norms and health-care utilization in highly religious, heterosexual men. Am J Men's Health 2019;13(3). https://doi.org/10.1177/1557988319856739. 155798831985673.

12. Wackerbarth JJ, Fantus RJ, Darves-Bornoz A, et al. Examining online traffic patterns to popular direct-to-consumer websites for evaluation and treatment of erectile Dysfunction. Sex Med 2021;9(1):100289.

13. Oster, PhD, MPH NV, Skillman, MS SM, Frogner, PhD BK. COVID-19's effect on the employment status of health care workers. FamilyMedicine.uw.edu. family medicine.uw.edu/chws/wp-content/uploads/sites/5/2021/05/ Health_Employ_Status_PB_May_26_2021.pdf. Published May 2021. Accessed February 28, 2023.

14. Bhasin S, Cunningham GR, Hayes FJ, et al. Testosterone therapy in men with androgen deficiency syndromes: an Endocrine Society clinical practice guideline. J Clin Endocrinol Metab 2010;95(6):2536–59.

15. Auerbach JM, Moghalu OI, Das R, et al. Evaluating incidence, prevalence, and treatment trends in adult men with hypogonadism in the United States. Int J Impot Res 2021. https://doi.org/10.1038/s41443-021-00471-2.

16. Ugo-Neff G, Rizzolo D. Hypogonadism in men. J Am Acad Physician Assist 2022; 35(5):28–34.

17. Calogero AE, Cannarella R, Agarwal A, et al. The renaissance of male infertility management in the golden age of andrology. The World Journal of Men's Health 2023;41. https://doi.org/10.5534/wjmh.220213.

18. Babakhanzadeh E, Nazari M, Ghasemifar S, et al. Some of the factors involved in male infertility: a prospective review. Int J Gen Med 2020;13:29–41.

19. Sharma KL, Alom M, Trost L. The etiology of peyronie's disease: pathogenesis and genetic contributions. Sexual Medicine Reviews 2020;8(2):314–23.

20. Ziegelmann MJ, Bajic P, Levine LA. Peyronie's disease: contemporary evaluation and management. Int J Urol 2020. https://doi.org/10.1111/iju.14230.

21. Langan RC. Benign Prostatic Hyperplasia. Prim Care Clin Office Pract 2019; 46(2):223–32.

22. Laumann EO, Glasser DB, Neves RCS, et al. A population-based survey of sexual activity, sexual problems and associated help-seeking behavior patterns in mature adults in the United States of America. Int J Impot Res 2009;21(3):171–8.

23. Census Results - American Urological Association. Available at: www.auanet.org. https://www.auanet.org/research/data-services/aua-census/census-results. Accessed March 1, 2023.

24. Tharakan T, Jayasena C, Minhas S. Men's health clinics: a real need or a marketing strategy. Int J Impot Res 2020;32(6):565–8.

25. Lipshultz LI, Pastuszak AW. Men's health: a rapidly changing landscape of healthcare delivery and treatment. Transl Androl Urol 2020;9(S2):S114–5.

26. Weinstein RS, Holcomb MJ, Krupinski EA, et al. First trainees: the golden anniversary of the early history of telemedicine education at the massachusetts general hospital and harvard (1968–1970). Telemedicine, Telehealth and Telepresence 2020;3–18. https://doi.org/10.1007/978-3-030-56917-4_1.

27. Robeznieks A. Which medical specialties use telemedicine the most? American Medical Association. Published January 11, 2019. Available at: https://www.ama-assn.org/practice-management/digital/which-medical-specialties-use-telemedicine-most. Accessed February 25, 2023.

28. Badalato GM, Kaag M, Lee R, et al. Role of telemedicine in urology: contemporary practice patterns and future directions. Urology Practice 2020;7(2):122–6.

29. Lucas JW, Villarroel MA. Telemedicine use among adults: United States, 2021. NCHS data brief 2022;(445):1–8. Available at: https://pubmed.ncbi.nlm.nih.gov/36255940/. Accessed March 1, 2023.
30. Dubin JM, Wyant WA, Balaji NC, et al. Telemedicine usage among urologists during the COVID-19 pandemic: cross-sectional study. J Med Internet Res 2020; 22(11):e21875.
31. Rabinowitz MJ, Kohn TP, Ellimoottil C, et al. The impact of telemedicine on sexual medicine at a major academic center during the COVID-19 pandemic. Sex Med 2021;9(3):100366.
32. Dorsey ER, Okun MS, Bloem BR. Care, convenience, comfort, confidentiality, and contagion: the 5 C's that will shape the future of telemedicine. J Parkinsons Dis 2020;10(3):893–7.
33. Miller A, Rhee E, Gettman M, et al. The current state of telemedicine in urology. Medical Clinics 2018;102(2):387–98.
34. Gajarawala S, Pelkowski J. Telehealth benefits and barriers. J Nurse Pract 2020; 17(2):218–21.
35. Dubin JM, Fantus RJ, Halpern JA. Testosterone replacement therapy in the era of telemedicine. Int J Impot Res 2021;34(7):663–8.
36. Demaerschalk BM, Cassivi SD, Blegen RN, et al. Health economic analysis of postoperative video telemedicine visits to patients' homes. Telemedicine and e-Health 2020. https://doi.org/10.1089/tmj.2020.0257.
37. Mulhall JP, Trost LW, Brannigan RE, et al. Evaluation and management of testosterone deficiency: AUA guideline. J Urol 2018;200(2):423–32.
38. Carter HB, Albertsen PC, Barry MJ, et al. Early detection of prostate cancer: AUA guideline. J Urol 2013;190(2):419–26.
39. Weinstein RS, Krupinski EA, Doarn CR. Clinical examination component of telemedicine, telehealth, mHealth, and connected health medical practices. Med Clin 2018;102(3):533–44.
40. Dooley AB, Houssaye N de la, Baum N. Use of telemedicine for sexual medicine patients. Sexual Medicine Reviews 2020;8(4):507–17.

# Testicular Cancer
## The Unmet Needs of a Younger Generation of Cancer Survivors

Blake K. Smith, MSN, BS, RN,[a,b,c,*]

### KEYWORDS

• Testicular cancer • Unmet needs • Survivorship • Men's health • Cancer support

### KEY POINTS

• Testicular Cancer Survivors face unique unmet societal, physical, emotional/psychological, and support needs.
• Gender identification of the testicular cancer survivor impacts success post-diagnosis.
• Providing education for males to understand is essential to avoid the knowledge deficit of the testicular cancer survivor.
• Societal factors play a significant role in how young men view themselves with a testicular cancer diagnosis.

▶ Video content accompanies this article at http://www.nursing.theclinics.com.

### Intro

Unmet holistic needs of various cancer populations, with examples including prostate, bladder, gynecologic, kidney, penile, breast, and colorectal, along with holistic impacts of cancer on older adults, have been defined by a growing number of systematic reviews (**Fig. 1**, Video 1). Unfortunately, there continues to be a lack of clinical insight into the unique needs of younger men with testicular cancer.[1] Testicular cancer is the 26th most commonly diagnosed cancer worldwide.[2] It is also the most prevalent type of cancer found in men ages 15 to 35, with 74,458 cases globally diagnosed in 2020.[3] Survival rate based on low mortality rates and good prognosis if early detection and treatment implementation grows the number of men who need support as long-term survivors with an average life expectancy of approximately 30 to 50 years after treatment.[4,5]

[a] American Association for Men in Nursing, Wisconsin Rapids, WI, USA; [b] Enterprise Applications, Nebraska Medicine, Omaha, NE, USA; [c] School of Nursing, Nebraska Methodist College, Omaha, NE, USA
* American Association for Men in Nursing, Wisconsin Rapids, WI.
*E-mail address:* blake.smithrn2012@gmail.com

Nurs Clin N Am 58 (2023) 581–593
https://doi.org/10.1016/j.cnur.2023.07.005
0029-6465/23/© 2023 Elsevier Inc. All rights reserved.

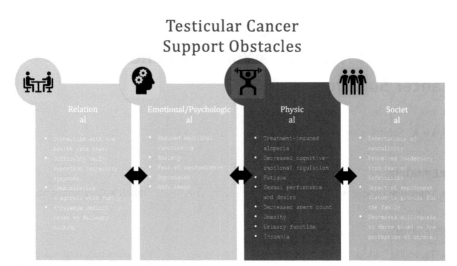

**Fig. 1.** Unmet Support Needs of Testicular Cancer Survivors.

Individual studies have found that due to the long life expectancy, the rate of testicular cancer survivors has led to an increased prevalence of distress, anxiety, depression, and fear of recurrence in testicular cancer survivors compared to other cancer and general populations.[4] Long-lasting effects from testicular cancer treatment include infertility, altered neurologic and respiratory function, procuring life insurance and employment, psychological distress (ie, fear of cancer recurrence), altered masculinity/body image, concerns with alopecia from chemotherapy, and challenges of intimacy and relationships.[6] These concerns and challenges have led to suicide, affected cognitive ability, and general fatigue when not addressed.[7] Additional holistic challenges include the self-regulation of managing the expectation of 5 a "cancer survivor" at a young age and the increased risk of being unable to move on with their lives.[8] The inability to successfully navigate into adulthood following cancer treatment frequently results in more significant functional challenges in later life.[7]

## TREATMENT CONSIDERATIONS

Testicular cancer is one of the most curable cancers, with a survival rate of 90%, primarily based on platinum-based chemotherapies.[9] Survivors must have a long-term follow-up for fertility and potentially developing secondary cancers, hypogonadism, sexual dysfunction, cardiovascular disease, metabolic syndrome, ongoing fatigue, and other concerns.[1] Several studies have found that treatments for testicular cancer, including surgery (orchiectomy), chemotherapy, and radiotherapy, can damage the reproductive organs resulting in sexual, social, and emotional dysfunction.[7] Chemotherapy increasingly deteriorates sexual life, while surgery significantly impacts intercourse and overall sexual satisfaction during recovery.[10] Stage I seminoma patients are candidates for surveillance, adjuvant carboplatin, or adjuvant after orchiectomy. Early detection and diagnosis are favorable as stage I treatment recommends surveillance after orchiectomy. Adjunctive radiotherapy and carboplatin-based chemotherapy are less preferred alternatives.[11] Treatment side effects are more significant in those who receive chemotherapy.[1] Surveillance is associated with the lowest risk of short-term and long-term treatment-related morbidity, with 80% of patients not experiencing recurrence and being cured with orchiectomy alone.

Testicular microlithiasis in the absence of a solid mass and risk factors for the development of germ cell tumor (GCT) does not represent an increased risk of malignant neoplasm. Therefore, the recommended treatment for further evaluation is not required.[1] Risk factors requiring closer evaluation include cryptorchidism, family history, personal history of GCT, or Germ Cell Neoplasia In Situ (GCNIS).[11] Additional treatments that include adjuvant carboplatin and radiation reduce reoccurrence but do not improve survival compared to surveillance post-orchiectomy alone.[11] Patients who receive chemotherapy have the most increased chance of experiencing a decreased Health-related Quality of Life (HRQOL) soon after treatment.[12]

## SOCIETAL CONSIDERATIONS

Adjustment to the testicular cancer experience is impacted by social aspects, including having children and marital and employment status.[4] Individuals who found themselves in good health with a perception of currently having a good life found the experience was an opportunity to make positive improvements in their lives.[13] Those with employed partners who had children and did not have a chronic disease were more likely to perceive their post-cancer experience positively.[14] Men's health includes applying social and cultural constructions that shape health behaviors and outcomes. However, there is less understanding of specific social-biological pathways based on gendered arrangements and how they embody differences among men compared to traditionally defined binary males and females. When providing care for those with testicular cancer, it is critical to recognize that socially defined categories, including gender, depend on one another to define these categories' meaning.[15]

Men's sexuality and gender identity are central to their notion of masculinity. Men's health and outcomes will be incomplete and biased if the provider fails to consider how gender intersects with other identities. Understanding the individual's culture is essential as it underpins men's conceptions about manhood.[7] Male individuals, defined by the presence of male reproductive organs, affected by testicular cancer reported needing assistance with their sexuality and sex life because they were embarrassed to discuss this with their health care provider.[16] Some are frustrated at not being able to maintain the role of a strongman in their relationship, exemplifying the need for some men to continue to display a notion of sexual prowess and stoicism. However, this is not the case for all men, with a study determining that men display feelings of sensitivity, modesty, curiosity, and vulnerability when affected by cancer.[17] The same study found clinicians stereotypically characterized male patients as disinterested, impatient, and stoic. It is essential for clinicians not to cast all men in the same light.[7]

### Relationships/Sexuality

Young men are associated with projecting a tough and emotionless persona that can lead to poorer health outcomes, especially in cases involving sensitive topics that include their genitals. The fault of these societal interactions with their environment lies in cultural influences that men place on each other.[7] There is a correlation in testicular cancer survivors that express a degree of distress due to the perception of themselves by others, which leads to not sharing their diagnosis.[13] Fertility serves as a determinant of men's sense of identity as partners, with one example including those who are the only male in the family having a sense of pressure to marry.[13] Information men received about long-term fertility issues confronted them suddenly and seriously.[18] Testicular cancer survivors significantly expressed more concern about fertility than men without the presence of the disease. However, testicular cancer survivors were more likely to report the distress and ask for infertility testing, though they were less likely to father children.[19] Survivors with nonseminoma expressed more significant overall distress about their inability to father children. Also, those men who perceived their attractiveness decreased after treatment were much more likely to experience significantly more symptoms of distress than those who perceived themselves as equally or more attractive before treatments.[7]

Testicular cancer survivors and their caregivers indicated that cancer made their social relationships difficult, and they wanted help and advice on creating new relationships with intimate partners.[7] Men were embarrassed to disclose concerns about the signs and symptoms of testicular cancer and apprehension about sharing their diagnosis with the people in their lives.[20] This difficulty brought forth reports of men wanting the availability to speak with other men who have gone through the same experience as they felt more comfortable being vulnerable among other survivors.[8] Men who were single/unmarried/un-partnered were more susceptible to a higher frequency and severity of the fear of recurrence than survivors who were married/partnered or had a robust support system in place. Problems within intimate relationships also surfaced because some participants felt they could not speak to their partner about sexual issues, which decreased general satisfaction with their sexual life and relationship.[1]

Testicular cancer survivor relationships with the health care team also are essential, with many individuals expressing the quality of care over telehealth being suboptimal compared to in-person consultations, especially during the COVID-19 pandemic. Caregivers and family members also felt isolated because they could not attend visits, support the patient during treatment, or be present during discussions with the medical team due to COVID-19 restrictions. The men who experienced procedures within the hospital felt isolated due to the visitor restrictions during their cancer journey though they were much less likely to report their isolation.[21]

### Social Determinants of Health

Males with testicular cancer also worry about other common life challenges that affect young and middle-aged life, including career impacts and body image.[4] These challenges can lead to a hopeless coping style and a cancer-related masculinity threat.[22] Those who describe economic and career concerns express anxiety and distress from their inability to work and insecurity of possible job loss.[18] Negative body image concerns are reported by those who feel a sense of decreased attractiveness after treatment and have experienced more stress-related symptoms.[7] Depression is more familiar with unmarried/lower social support, fatigue, adverse health behaviors, avoidant and helpless/hopeless coping, poorer sexual functioning, previous psychological distress, altered body image, and a sense of masculinity.[4] These perceived social constructs to emotional disclosure might negatively affect men's adjustment to cancer.[23] Others alluded to medical insurance or reimbursement issues, loss of employment, financial difficulties, reduced working hours or being forced to take sick or annual leave. People affected by cancer also shared worries concerning job security, the disruption this causes to daily functioning, and broader family-related needs. Patients sacrificed their self-care due to work demands. Few participated in exercise or health self-management behaviors.[21]

Race (and ethnicity) remains a valuable marker of exposure to health-harming environments and substances, social disadvantage, and health-promoting resources.[15] Unemployed men had significantly more unmet needs than those employed.[7] Singles, those with less education, and those without employment had higher cancer-related stress symptoms.[24] The fact that some racial (and ethnic) groups are more likely to live in poverty, work in low-paying and dangerous occupations, reside in closer proximity to polluted environments, be exposed to toxic substances, experience threats and realities of crime, and live with cumulative concerns about meeting basic needs highlights the importance of considering both gendered and non-gendered aspects of their environments, identities, and experiences.[15] Testicular cancer survivors who are not employed, have lower educational status, and are single are at higher risk of elevated distress.[4] Current studies strongly correlate that the physical needs among testicular cancer survivors are associated with unemployment, age, low socioeconomic status, and anxiety and depression.[25] While there are similarities in the practical needs identified in broader cancer care literature, there is much more concern about work, school, and finances in this young population than in older adults.[26] Understanding the poor status of men's health and premature death includes considering how racialized and gendered social determinants of health shape men's lives and experiences, mainly through economic and environmental factors.[15]

## PHYSICAL IMPLICATIONS

Physical needs are prevalent in testicular cancer survivors, who, on average, may experience 4.5 physical symptoms (SD = 4.4; range, 1–28).[7] Cancer of a sexual organ leads to concerns and challenges around meeting certain sexual and masculine stereotypes at a young age and may cause symptoms of depression.[4] Testicular cancer survivors have lower mean vitality, physical functioning, physical role functioning, and general health compared to the general healthy population.[1] Men had physical concerns related to having one testicle, which relates to psychological consequences and intimacy concerns, including those who elected prostheses and were unhappy with the aesthetic result.[16] Those who reported the most favorable health reported changes in their body image after orchidectomy only with surveillance or with the addition of adjuvant radiotherapy.[8] Other general physical well-being experienced disturbances in sleep, eating, and exercise.[21]

### Physical Symptoms

Most commonly, testicular cancer survivors experience fatigue, lack of energy, drowsiness, pain, hair loss, and sleep disturbances. Other less commonly experience symptoms but still cause distress among testicular cancer survivors including itching, cough, sweats, shortness of breath, dizziness, skin changes, mucositis, numbness, tingling, bloated, and changed taste, urination difficulties, diarrhea, and constipation.[25] Obesity is also a determinant of these late effects, and thus lifestyle behaviors, such as smoking, drinking, and low physicality, may be linked to long-term health conditions post-treatment.[24]

The cancer treatment can drive physical symptoms, the most common being fatigue. It could also be driven by societal impacts, such as financial difficulties leading to insomnia which significantly affects the health-related quality of life of the individual.[7] Chemotherapy side-effects related to cognitive function seem to be associated with higher distress.[4] Men also grappled with chemotherapy-induced alopecia and reported needing help with hair loss. However, preventative strategies for alopecia, such as scalp cooling, are inconsistently addressed.[1] The lack of energy and tiredness is exhibited as temper outbursts or frustration from the lack of control of the situation.[21] If these physical symptoms are recognized and treated alongside cancer, they will present only temporarily. Once treatment has concluded, the individual returns to a similar state before treatment.[13]

### Sexual Performance Impact

Sexual problems seriously affect the quality of life in testicular cancer survivors and are not dependent on treatment type or significance.[7] Intimacy needs are high for patient populations where cancer affects the reproductive organs or secondary sexual characteristics, which can negatively impact the sexuality of the affected person.[27] A recent study found that at least 26% of patients with testicular cancer experienced sexual dysfunction, and 28% had significant reproductive concerns.[4] The most commonly experienced issues for these young men included erectile dysfunction, reduced erectile rigidity, and inability to maintain an erection during intercourse due to chronic pain.[28–30] Additionally, problems with fertility, hypogonadism, higher white matter hyperintensities, radial kurtosis, and low testosterone were reported.[31] Significantly reduced libido, lower intensity of orgasm, and difficulties in maintaining erections are reported in patients with seminoma treated with radiotherapy.[32] Another review determined that although sperm counts were initially lower in testicular cancer survivors, counts had normalized when reassessed 5 years later.[7] Some men had a lower sexual desire and erectile dysfunction three to 5 years following therapy completion.[33] Evidence from some studies by Kim and colleagues[34] reported a decrease in sexual function, erectile dysfunction, and a loss of desire. In the case-control study, survivors experienced more significant impairment or dysfunction than controls, with sexual dysfunction varied by treatment modality. The authors found that combined chemotherapy and surgery treatment showed a greater risk of decreased libido or ejaculatory dysfunction. In contrast, a combination of radiation and surgical treatment was more closely associated with erectile dysfunction.[34]

## EMOTIONAL/PSYCHOLOGICAL IMPLICATIONS

Overall, studies reported negative impacts on mental health, reduced emotional functioning, low mental component summary scores, and reduced emotional vitality.[1] Stress, anxiety, depression, fear of recurrence, and body image issues were commonly experienced.[8,35] One study showed that at least 20% of testicular cancer survivors needed psychological support due to the cancer experience even after 7 to 10 years post-treatment.[4]

Cognitive-Emotional Regulation relates to distress in testicular cancer survivors.[4] Evidence identified that as many as 58% of testicular cancer survivors could experience cognitive impairment, which is significant given this young cohort of men who could be either studying or working in paid employment.[36] Emotional needs are related to emotional functioning and depression.[37] Individuals reported significantly poorer overall mental health for testicular cancer survivors and a higher prevalence of moderate to extremely severe anxiety and depression than the general population.[7] Testicular Cancer survivors reported that they were embarrassed about a loss of maleness and expressed fears about how to hold onto their self-esteem.[18] Many participants described that they had come to terms with living with cancer but were afraid and experienced anxiety and a sense of a lack of control.[21] One study identified that faith and the meaning of life were rated as least concerning unmet needs, and testicular cancer survivors reported that they had no unmet spiritual needs in this young patient group, but in many instances may not be accurate due to the lack of discussion of the topic with young men.[1]

### Emotional Considerations

Testicular cancer survivors experience a higher severity of distress than the general male population in a multivariable-adjusted analysis regardless of treatment received.

One in three testicular cancer survivors suffers from fear of cancer recurrence, with studies reporting between 37% and 58% of survivors experiencing above-threshold levels of fear of recurrence, as well as single men found to report less fear of recurrence than partnered men.[4] Men also described a fear of the unknown, a fear of the future, and a fear of dying.[18] Survivors had a higher prevalence of distress than the general male population until the age of 70 (after this age, the general population becomes more distressed). Participants in several studies discussed how they struggled with the emotional fallout of their disease, with one participant expressing sadness and frustration at not being able to maintain the "strong" role in his relationship with his girlfriend.[7] One study reported that the surgical removal of the testicle and waiting for X-ray results caused intense fear, while illness resulting from chemotherapy caused feelings of helplessness.[24] During the COVID-19 pandemic, these fears increased to include the long-term impact that the pandemic would have on treatment outcomes, care follow-up, clinical service delays, and the overall impact that this would have on them in the future.[21]

The impacts of these emotional aspects of cancer treatment and its side effects prevented some men from returning to work in one study, with a participant experiencing an emotional breakdown and taking time off work. Others experienced being unable to fully understand and express emotions, nervousness, tension, sadness, restlessness, and sleep problems.[7] Spiritual support is also significantly lacking. This may represent a deficient holistic assessment that leads to further support during difficult times based on assumptions of young men and their relations to spirituality.[7] The importance of addressing the emotional needs of those experiencing testicular cancer treatment is that positive outcomes can occur for those provided with appropriate support reporting the most frequently mentioned changes were more appreciative of life, enjoying life more, a more conscious experience, and appreciation of the here and now, seeing things in a different perspective, a re-evaluation of priorities and reprioritization of what is essential in life.[14]

### Psychological Considerations

Testicular cancer survivors report a higher prevalence and severity of anxiety than the general population. There is also evidence that the younger the patient, the higher the risk of experiencing clinical anxiety levels. Anxiety was not age dependent among patients with testicular cancer, as it has shown between those with cancer and the general population without cancer. Survivors may experience more significant anxiety due to the existential challenge to their sense of invulnerability posed by being diagnosed with a life-threatening illness at a relatively young age.[4] Age is associated with depressive symptoms in another study where younger cancer survivors reported more significant depressive symptoms than older cancer survivors.[23] This correlation is similar to anxiety as it is not age-related or a significant difference between treatment types among testicular cancer survivors. Qualitative and quantitative studies have reported a renewed appreciation for life and a more positive outlook after testicular cancer with decreased depression prevalence. These findings are cautioned as the commonly used measures of depression (eg, the HADS-D) do not assess externalizing depressive symptoms (eg, substance misuse, risk-taking, and poor impulse control) and present more frequently and with greater intensity in men versus women with depression.[4]

Testicular cancer survivors are often concerned about sexuality, fertility, body image, and male identity, which can impact survivors' quality of life.[4] Body image concerns are associated with sexual dysfunction in testicular cancer survivors.[38] Similarly, there were feelings of a distorted body image and loss of attractiveness in testicular cancer survivors, and less frequent sexual activity was significantly related to more significant stress.[7] However, it is unlikely that all sexual dysfunction reported in this review is only attributed to a psychogenic nature, given the consistently high rates of sexual dysfunction in the testicular cancer survivor populations.[39] One individual's statement on sexual and body image was as follows:

> 'It just feels kind of like you're incomplete. Just as a person you feel like you're missing something you're supposed to have. I guess it's just the fact that it doesn't have any real effect, but there's still something missing. So it's just that weird dichotomy' (Participant 9)" (page 742).[20]

## SUPPORT NEEDS

Supportive care is a holistic term that describes a person-centered approach to delivering oncology services for individuals diagnosed with cancer to meet their informational, spiritual, psychological, social, or physical needs across the cancer care continuum.[6] Addressing supportive care needs is the foundation of a successful intervention because of its positive influence on the quality of life and psychosocial outcomes.[21] Fundamental gaps in information for knowledge and understanding of which treatments men received, the associated risks of treatments, lifestyle advice to support self-management within the multidisciplinary team, timely access to results, and how to self-report concerning symptoms to health care professionals are reported by survivors.[1]

### Caregiver Participation and Engagement

People diagnosed with cancer needed to have their family or support network at their side as a critical psychosocial aspect of care; however, during the pandemic, this recently was not allowed.[21] Young men expressed a need to know how to support their partners or families, how to communicate with their young children, and concerns about being unable to have children due to fertility issues.[1] Being fertile, having children, and living with a partner were essential aspects of good health-related quality of life. Men employed full-time and men living with a partner reported more positive effects.[7] Studies have found that married patients or those in a stable relationship cope better with cancer than unmarried patients or single patients, possibly related to the cultural norms of that society.[40] For those who lacked family support during consultations, leads to a significant change in opportunities that contributed to decisional regret in cancer treatment and care decision-making.[21] These findings show the importance of better supporting testicular cancer survivors' caregivers to optimize outcomes for survivors and their caregivers, as greater social support is associated with better psychological outcomes.[4]

### Health Care Team Relationship

Men expressed that they wanted to feel more supported in the self-management of their health in partnership with their health care team.[1] A problem cited by men in some studies was the need for more information they received about the effects of surgery and the inability of oncologists to provide enough time to have the right conversations.[41] Many of the men in one study felt that their oncologists did not have enough time to provide information and reassurance about these issues, which resulted in men expressing frustration about not being able to have the right conversations even when they tried to initiate them.[7] One study conducted during the COVID-19 pandemic led to the transition of utilizing telehealth similarly restricted opportunities to engage with health care professionals. Some participants noted a change in empathy and an attitude toward blaming COVID-19 for everything that went wrong.[21] The communication aspects found to be most impactful to these young men were an appropriate tone used by health professionals. They included sensitive language, a positive, helpful approach, a respectful manner, and the use of humor to normalize the illness. In addition, men consistently reported that receiving honest, straightforward information was helpful.[7]

### Knowledge Deficit and Education Delivery

Noteworthy, 50% of testicular cancer survivors did not know what information supports were available to them.[1] Individuals affected by testicular cancer reported needing help with their sex life because they were embarrassed to discuss this with health care professionals.[8] Similarly, in another study, most survivors wished they had received information about everyday stress and crisis reactions and been offered professional counseling.[41] Men also wanted information on how to access complementary or alternative therapies and information on sexual recovery.[1] Testicular cancer survivors have described not being provided with comprehensive information on what to expect post-treatment, with many instructed to "adapt" and return to their "normal" lives. This approach made the patient feel it was up to them to seek their information without the support of the health care team.[7]

This perceived lack of communication and education from the health care team on the availability of information and resources results from a misunderstanding of how men receive information and learn. One of the most common unmet needs reported in another study concerned men's identities as cancer survivors, suggesting a lack of psychosocial and practical support.[7] A review of 37 men's depression help-seeking studies found that strength-and courage-based masculine norms could promote help-seeking and that men prefer collaborative interventions involving action-oriented problem-solving. Endorsement by testicular cancer survivors of sport-based approaches with embedded psychoeducation have the added benefit of providing additional social support, which is associated with better outcomes.[4]

## DISCUSSION

Patients with cancer report physical, psychological/emotional, cognitive, patient-clinician communication, health system/information, spiritual, daily living, interpersonal/intimacy, practical, family, and social needs.[21] Men suffer psychologically from testicular cancer experiences if they cannot meet the standard of masculinity set by prevalent cultural narratives. Anxiety is the primary psychological burden for testicular cancer, with depression, fear of cancer recurrence, and distress seeming less prevalent and severe.[4] Further evidence of higher distress levels in testicular cancer survivors who are unemployed, unmarried (as in the general population), or with poor self-assessed fitness, but specific aspects of the diagnosis and treatment of TC (eg, treatment type), were unrelated to distress. While distress seems more common in testicular cancer survivors than in the general population, there is currently little additional evidence regarding the correlation of distress related explicitly to the experience of testicular cancer.[4]

More efforts are needed to determine patient characteristics that increase the risk of higher anxiety scores. One small fair-quality study found anxiety was associated with sexual confidence, functioning, and cognitive-emotion regulation. More research is also needed to understand how testicular cancer survivors' psychological outcomes impact partners' or caregivers' well-being and ability to provide support. It is also noteworthy that the men represented one of few systematic reviews that did not express concerns with existential issues or fear of death and dying, commonly experienced in other cancer populations. It would be essential to explore whether these were concealed concerns because of their age or reticence to disclose, but ultimately this remains unknown.[1]

### Application of Intervention

Techniques such as latent class analysis may help identify the factors that differentiate the minority of testicular cancer survivors who experience poorer outcomes from the majority who adjust well. Given that testicular cancer impacts male lives, supporting men throughout the trajectory is prudent. Using Kanker Nazorg Wijzer's intervention could be an invaluable theory-based, wide-ranging web resource for providing support to cancer survivors, including those men surviving testicular cancer.[42] There is a pressing need to identify testicular cancer survivors who require psychological support and may benefit from the growing number of psychological interventions for testicular cancer survivors.[4] Age was a significant risk factor for depression for overall cancer survivors, where the mean age for patients was 35.5 years. Testicular cancer impacts young men at the mean average or below, increasing the need for offering them options to reduce anxiety through self-management or consultation with an allied health professional is recommended.[7] The correlation of depression in testicular cancer survivors, such as threats to masculinity, sexual difficulties, and maladaptive coping strategies, may not be immediately apparent or readily disclosed, so screening for depression may be warranted.[4] Cognitive behavioral therapy and educational programs can be leveraged to manage and reduce fatigue in survivors.[43]

Evidence has demonstrated that men affected by testicular cancer commonly report at least one unmet supportive care need despite routine clinical follow-ups.[16] Providers should focus on testicular cancer survivors and their families and caregivers, considering cultural differences, age, and the socioeconomic status during the communication episodes.[44] Assuring survivors of testicular cancer that the chances of fathering children are not significantly diminished post-treatment is essential, as this can impact their psychological well-being.[7] Issues encountered by these men were a lack of opportunity to discuss these problems with their intimate partner or health care professionals, often because of embarrassment.[1] Men who underwent orchidectomy were less affected mentally than those who underwent chemotherapy with surveillance or adjuvant radiotherapy. Survivors treated with chemotherapy reported lower emotional well-being than men with other treatment modalities, but the difference was insignificant.[7]

## SUMMARY

Testicular Cancer survivors are becoming more prevalent due to the advancements in treatment and early detection. Unmet needs continue to be inconsistent based on gaps in research and the ability to connect with the patient populations affected. Testicular cancer survivors continue to experience unique needs that are different from other types of cancer disease processes based on the impact of testicular cancer on societal, physical, and emotional/psychological needs to flourish as survivors. It is essential for providers and clinicians to approach testicular cancer survivors with the tools and strategies that meet these unmet needs for navigation from diagnosis through survivorship. When strategies of specific resources and education are implemented based on the unique needs of these individuals, positive outcomes and increased health care -related quality of life will be prevalent.

## CLINICS CARE POINTS

- Testicular Cancer is the most prevalent type of cancer found in men ages 15 to 35, with 74,458 cases globally diagnosed in 2020.
- Early detection and treatment implementation grows the number of men who need support as long-term survivors with an average life expectancy of approximately 30 to 50 years after treatment.
- Existing studies have reported enduring and long lasting effects from treatment which include problems related to infertility, altered neurological and respiratory function, problems in securing life insurance and employment, psychological distress (such as fear of cancer recurrence), altered masculinity/ body image, concerns related to chemotherapy-induced alopecia, and challenges with intimacy and relationships.
- Evidence has demonstrated that men affected by testicular cancer commonly report at least one unmet supportive care need despite routine clinical follow-up.

## DISCLOSURE

The author of this articles does not have any commercial or financial conflicts of interest in addition to not having any funding sources.

## SUPPLEMENTARY DATA

Supplementary data related to this article can be found online at https://doi.org/10.1016/j.cnur.2023.07.005.

## REFERENCES

1. Doyle R, Craft P, Turner M, et al. Identifying the unmet supportive care needs of individuals affected by testicular cancer: a systematic review. J Cancer Surviv 2022. https://doi.org/10.1007/s11764-022-01219-7.
2. Pishgar F, Haj-Mirzaian A, Ebrahimi H, et al. Global, regional and national burden of testicular cancer, 1990–2016: results from the Global Burden of Disease Study 2016. BJU Int 2019;124(3):386–94.
3. Znaor A, Skakkebæk NE, Rajpert-De Meyts E, et al. Testicular cancer incidence predictions in Europe 2010–2035: a rising burden despite population ageing. Int J Cancer 2020;147(3):820–8.
4. Rincones O, Allan'Ben'Smith SN, Mercieca-Bebber R, et al. An updated systematic review of quantitative studies assessing anxiety, depression, fear of cancer recurrence or psychological distress in testicular cancer survivors. Cancer Manag Res 2021;13:3803.
5. Shaikh AJ, Dhillion N, Shah J, et al. Supporting Kenyan women with advanced breast cancer through a network and assessing their needs and quality of life. Support Care Cancer 2022;30(2):1557–67.
6. Paterson C, Kozlovskaia M, Turner M, et al. Identifying the supportive care needs of men and women affected by chemotherapy-induced alopecia? A systematic review. J Cancer Surviv 2021;15(1):14–28.
7. Alexis O, Adeleye AO, Worsley AJ. Men's experiences of surviving testicular cancer: an integrated literature review. Journal of Cancer Survivorship 2020;14(3):284–93.

8. Batehup L, Gage H, Williams P, et al. Unmet supportive care needs of breast, colorectal and testicular cancer survivors in the first 8 months post primary treatment: a prospective longitudinal survey. Eur J Cancer Care 2021;30(6):e13499.

9. de Vries G, Rosas-Plaza X, van Vugt MA, et al. Testicular cancer: Determinants of cisplatin sensitivity and novel therapeutic opportunities. Cancer Treat Rev 2020; 88:102054.

10. Dimitropoulous K, Karatzas A, Papandreou C, et al. Sexual dysfunctional testicular cancer patients subjected to post-chemotherapy retroperitoneal lymph node dissection: a focus beyond ejaculation disorders. Andrologia 2016;48: 425–30.

11. Stephenson A, Eggener SE, Bass EB, et al. Diagnosis and treatment of early stage testicular cancer: AUA guideline. J Urol 2019;202(2):272–81.

12. Vidrine DJ, Hoekstra-Weebers JEHM, Hoekstra H, et al. The effects of testicular Cancer treatment on health-related quality of life. Urology 2010;75(3):636–41.

13. Saab M, Noureddine S, Huijer HA-S, et al. Surviving testicular Cancer: the Lebanese lived experience. Nurs Res 2014;63(3):203–10.

14. Fleer J, Hoekstra HJ, Sleijfer D, et al. The role of meaning in the prediction of psychosocial well-being of testicular cancer survivors. Qual Life Res 2006b;15: 705–17.

15. Griffith DM. An intersectional approach to men's health. J Mens Health 2012;9(2): 106–12.

16. Smith AB, King M, Butow P, et al. The prevalence and correlates of supportive care needs in testicular cancer survivors: a cross-sectional study. Psycho Oncol 2013;22(11):2557–64.

17. Soejima T, Kamibeppu K. Are cancer survivors well-performing workers? A systematic review. Asia Pac J Clin Oncol 2016;12:e383–97.

18. Kristjanson LJ, Ng C, Oldham L, et al. The impact and responses of men who have experienced testicular cancer. Aust J Cancer Nurs 2006;7(1):10–7.

19. Kim C, McGlynn KA, McCorkle R, et al. Fertility among testicular cancer survivors: a case-study in the U.S. J Cancer Surviv 2010;4:266–73.

20. Carpentier MY, Fortenberry JD, Ott MA, et al. Perceptions of masculinity and self-image in adolescent and young adult testicular cancer survivors: Implications for romantic and sexual relationships. Psycho Oncol 2011;20(7):738–45.

21. Legge H, Toohey K, Kavanagh PS, et al. The unmet supportive care needs of people affected by cancer during the COVID-19 pandemic: an integrative review. Journal of Cancer Survivorship 2022;1–21.

22. Wang AW-T, Hoyt MA. Cancer-related masculinity threat in young adults with testicular cancer the moderating role of benefit finding. Hist Philos Logic 2020; 33(2):207–15.

23. Thornton CP. Best practice in teaching male adolescents and young men to perform testicular self examinations: a review. J Pediatr Health Care 2016; 30(6):518–27.

24. Fleer J, Sleijfer D, Hoekstra H, et al. Objective and subjective predictors of cancer-related stress symptoms in testicular cancer survivors. Patient Educ Couns 2006c;64:142–50.

25. Oechsle K, Hartmann M, Mehnert A, et al. Symptom burden in long-term germ cell tumor survivors. Support Care Cancer 2016;24(5):2243–50.

26. Tracy JK, Falk D, Thompson RJ, et al. Managing the cancer-work interface: the effect of cancer survivorship on unemployment. Cancer Manag Res 2018;10: 6479–87.

27. Maleki M, Mardani A, Ghafourifard M, et al. Qualitative exploration of sexual life among breast cancer survivors at reproductive age. BMC Wom Health 2021; 21(1):56.
28. Kerns SL, Fung C, Fossa SD, et al. Relationship of cisplatin-related adverse health outcomes with disability and unemployment among testicular cancer survivors. JNCI Cancer Spectr 2020;4(4):022.
29. Pühse G, JU Wachsmuth, Kemper S, et al. Chronic pain has a negative impact on sexuality in testis cancer survivors. J Androl 2012;33(5):886–93.
30. Soleimani M, Kollmannsberger C, Bates A, et al. Patient-reported psychosocial distress in adolescents and young adults with germ cell tumours. Support Care Cancer 2021;29(4):2105–10.
31. De Padova S, Rosti G, Scarpi E, et al. Expectations of survivors, caregivers and healthcare providers for testicular cancer survivorship and quality of life. Tumori Journal 2011;97(3):367–73.
32. Capogrosso P, Boeri L, Ferrari M. Long-term recovery of normal sexual function in testicular cancer survivors. Asian J Andrology 2016;18:85–9.
33. Eberhard J, Stahl O, Cohn-Cedermark G, et al. Sexual function in men treated for testicular cancer. J Sex Med 2009;6(7):1979–89.
34. Kim C, McGlynn KA, McCorkle R, et al. Sexual functioning among testicular cancer survivors: a case-control study in the U.S. J Psychosom Res 2012;73(1): 68–73.
35. O'Carrigan B, Fournier M, Olver I, et al. Testosterone deficiency and quality of life in A ustralasian testicular cancer survivors: a prospective cohort study. Intern Med J 2014;44(8):813–7.
36. Amidi A, Wu LM, Agerbæk M, et al. Cognitive impairment and potential biological and psychological correlates of neuropsychological performance in recently orchiectomized testicular cancer patients. Psycho Oncol 2015;24(9):1174–80.
37. Alacacioglu A, Ulger E, Varol U, et al. Sexual satisfaction, anxiety, depression and quality of life in testicular cancer survivors. Med Oncol 2014;31(7):1–6.
38. Rossen P, Pedersen AF, Zachariae R, et al. Sexuality and body image in long-term survivors of testicular cancer. Eur J Cancer 2012;48(4):571–8.
39. La Vignera S, Cannarella R, Duca Y, et al. Hypogonadism and sexual dysfunction in testicular tumor survivors: a systematic review. Front Endocrinol 2019;10:264.
40. Lee TK, Handy AB, Kwan W, et al. Impact of prostate cancer treatment on the sexual quality of life for men-who-have-sex-with-men. J Sex Med 2015;12: 2378–86.
41. Skoogh J, Steineck G, Johansson B, et al, SWENOTECA. Psychological needs when diagnosed with testicular cancer: findings from a population-based study with long-term follow-up. BJU Int 2013;111:1287–93.
42. Kanera IM, Bolman CAW, Willems RA, et al. Lifestyle related effects of the web-based Kanker Nazorg Wijzer (cancer aftercare guide) intervention for cancer survivors: a randomized controlled trial. J Cancer Surviv 2016;10:883–97.
43. Cappuccio F, Rossetti S, Cavaliere C, et al. HRQoL and psychosocial implications in testicular cancer survivors. A literature review. Eur Rev Med Pharmacol Sci 2018;22(3):645–61.
44. De Padova S, Casadei C, Berardi A, et al. Caregiver emotional burden in testicular cancer patients: from patient to caregiver support. Front Endocrinol 2019; 10(318):1–7.

# Consideration of Gender in Cardiovascular Disease Prevention and Management

Kathleen M. Elertson, DNP, APNP, CPNP-PC, FNP-BC*,
Lindsay L. Morgan, DNP, APNP, FNP-BC

## KEYWORDS

- Heart disease • Biological sex and gender differences • Prevention • Management

## KEY POINTS

- Gender affects the clinical presentation of heart disease. Heart disease in women remains undermanaged.
- Providers are more likely to attribute cardiac concerns to other conditions in women compared with men.
- Reporting and presentation of symptoms by gender should be considered in the management and prevention of heart disease.

## INTRODUCTION

Gender-specific health care has emerged as a crucial aspect in the prevention and management of heart disease. Cardiovascular disease (CVD) is one of the leading causes of death among men and women globally.[1] CVD is multifactorial, resulting from a complex interplay of genetic, environmental, and lifestyle factors. Research has shown the prevalence, diagnosis, and management of heart disease differs between men and women. Although heart disease is sometimes considered to be a male-focused condition, mortalities are almost equal between men and women in the United States. Gender studies have noted women have lower rates of CVD; however, they are also more likely to die from a cardiac event compared with their male counterparts.[2] Identifying gender differences in CVD may improve prevention strategies, detection, and management in both men and women. In addition, biological sex-specific factors, such as hormonal differences, contribute to the pathophysiology, evaluation, and pharmacologic management of heart disease in men and women.[1,2] It

University of Wisconsin Oshkosh, College of Nursing, 800 Algoma Boulevard, Oshkosh, WI 54901, USA
* Corresponding author.
*E-mail address:* elertsok@uwosh.edu

is critical for health care providers to gain awareness of gender differences and risk factors to effectively address CVD.[2]

## BACKGROUND

Women tend to develop CVD later in life as compared with men and often present with atypical symptoms, creating a diagnostic challenge.[2] Moreover, women are less likely to receive appropriate medical management for their CVD, including guideline-recommended medications and interventions, resulting in poorer health outcomes.[3] To address this disparity, effective medical management of CVD requires tailored approaches that consider gender differences, including sex-specific screening, diagnostic tests, and treatment strategies. Bridging the CVD gender gap requires a multifaceted approach that involves comprehensive information gathering, gender-specific evidence-based best practices, enhanced research opportunities, and targeted education. Health care providers should increase awareness about the importance of cardiovascular health and take proactive measures to promote a healthy lifestyle within all populations.[1]

Coronary artery disease (CAD) is the most common form of CVD and occurs when there is a narrowing or blockage of the coronary arteries that supply blood to the heart. The primary mechanism underlying CAD is atherosclerosis, which involves the accumulation of cholesterol, inflammatory cells, and other substances in the arterial wall, leading to the formation of plaques that can obstruct blood flow and cause ischemia or infarction of the myocardium.[3] The development of CAD is a complex process involving multiple factors, including genetics, lifestyle, and environmental influences.[3] The risk factors for CAD include age, male sex, smoking, hypertension, dyslipidemia, diabetes mellitus, obesity, physical inactivity, and family history of premature CAD.[4] Men are more likely to develop CAD at a younger age compared with women. The incidence of CAD in men begins to increase in the third decade of life, whereas the incidence among women begins to increase after menopause.[2] The increased incidence of CAD in men has been attributed to a variety of factors, including differences in sex hormones, lifestyle factors, and genetic predisposition. Men are also more likely than women to smoke and have higher rates of obesity and physical inactivity, which may be contributing factors.[5]

Although prevalence of CAD is higher in men than in women, particularly in younger age groups, recent studies have shown that women are often misdiagnosed or underdiagnosed with heart disease, leading to delayed or inadequate treatment.[2,4] This difference in prevalence is partly attributed to the protective effect of estrogen in women, which has anti-inflammatory, antioxidant, and vasodilatory properties that reduce the risk of atherosclerosis.[2] After menopause, women lose the protective effect of estrogen, and their overall risk of CAD increases, approaching that of men of similar age.[3,4] Women tend to have more diffuse and less obstructive CAD than men, which may explain why they are less likely to present with typical angina symptoms, leading to a delay in diagnosis and treatment.[4]

Men tend to present with classic symptoms during an acute cardiovascular event, such as chest pain or discomfort. Women are more likely to present with atypical symptoms, such as shortness of breath, fatigue, or indigestion, which are often misinterpreted as anxiety or depression.[2,3] Women are also more likely to have other risk factors for CAD and may experience symptoms at rest.[5] Consequently, women are less likely to undergo diagnostic tests, such as electrocardiogram (ECG), stress tests, or coronary angiography, which are vital in the diagnosis of heart disease.[3,4] Another factor contributing to gender disparities in the medical management of

CAD is the underrepresentation of women in clinical trials. Historically, clinical trials have included male participants, with women often excluded owing to concerns about hormonal fluctuations and potential pregnancy.[2,4,5] This has resulted in a lack of evidence-based guidelines for the management of CVD in women. There have been targeted efforts for increased inclusion of women in clinical trials, with regulatory agencies such as the Food and Drug Administration requiring the inclusion of women in clinical trials.[3] This is a positive step toward addressing gender disparities in the medical management of CVD. In addition to the aforementioned factors, socioeconomic and cultural factors can also contribute to gender disparities in the medical management of CAD. Women from low-income backgrounds are more likely to have limited access to health care and are therefore less likely to receive timely and appropriate care.[1,2,4] Similarly, cultural factors can influence health care–seeking behavior, with women from certain cultures being less likely to seek medical attention or disclose symptoms related to CAD, which leads to underdiagnosis and undertreatment in these populations.[1,5,6]

Heart failure (HF) is a syndrome characterized by the impairment of the heart's ability to pump blood efficiently, leading to fluid retention, dyspnea, fatigue, and reduced exercise tolerance.[5] The pathophysiology of HF is complex and involves various mechanisms, such as myocardial damage, remodeling, and fibrosis, neurohormonal activation, inflammation, and oxidative stress. The risk factors for HF include age, male sex, hypertension, CAD, diabetes mellitus, obesity, smoking, and alcohol abuse.[5,7] The prevalence of HF is similar in men and women, but there are significant differences in the clinical presentation and outcomes between the sexes.[5] Although the overall management of HF is similar across different demographic groups, emerging evidence suggests that gender-specific approaches to CVD management are necessary.[3,5] It is essential to recognize these differences and tailor management strategies to meet gender-specific needs. By adopting an individualized approach to CVD management, health care professionals can optimize outcomes and improve overall quality of care for all patients.

## DISCUSSION
### Clinical Relevance

The evaluation of CVD includes a thorough medical history, physical examination, ECG, echocardiography, stress testing, and coronary angiography.[2,5] Men are more susceptible to atherosclerotic disease with significant coronary artery stenosis, whereas women are more likely to have microvascular disease and endothelial dysfunction.[8] In men, CAD is typically characterized by the presence of significant luminal stenosis in the coronary arteries, which leads to myocardial ischemia and angina pectoris. The underlying pathophysiology of CAD in men is often related to the presence of traditional risk factors, such as smoking, hypertension, dyslipidemia, and diabetes mellitus.[3,5,6,8] In men, a positive stress test or obstructive CAD on angiography may indicate a need for revascularization with percutaneous coronary intervention (PCI) or coronary artery bypass graft surgery.[5,8] In women, a normal stress test does not rule out the presence of microvascular disease. In women, CAD tends to be more diffuse and involves the microvascular levels of the heart. Women are more likely to have nonobstructive coronary artery disease (NOCAD), which is defined as less than 50% luminal stenosis on coronary angiography. Coronary arteries may appear normal during angiography despite having significant disease.[8] The underlying pathophysiology of NOCAD in women is complex and multifactorial and includes microvascular dysfunction, endothelial dysfunction, coronary artery spasm, and plaque erosion or rupture.[5,8] Moreover, women are more susceptible to adverse events after PCI owing to differences in vascular access, bleeding risk, and medication dosing.[8] Enhanced diagnostic testing with cardiac MRI or PET may be necessary.[5] Women also have unique risk factors, such as pregnancy-related complications, menopause, and autoimmune disorders, that can increase their risk of CVD.[2,3] It is important for health care providers to be aware of these differences and to consider CAD as a potential diagnosis in all patients, regardless of sex or age. Identification of modifiable risk factors, early recognition, and gender-specific evidence-based treatment of CAD can improve outcomes and reduce the risk of heart attack or stroke.[4]

Hypertension, or high blood pressure, is a major risk factor for heart disease in both men and women. However, the prevalence, control, and outcomes of hypertension differ between the sexes. About one-fifth of adults with hypertension remain undiagnosed.[7] In general, men have a higher prevalence of hypertension compared with women until the age of 65 years. However, after the age of 65 years, women have a higher prevalence of hypertension compared with men.[6,7] Women with hypertension are more likely to have isolated systolic hypertension, which is associated with an increased risk of CVD) events.[2] In addition, women with hypertension have a higher risk of developing left ventricular hypertrophy, which is a strong predictor of adverse cardiovascular outcomes.[5,8,9]

### Therapeutic Options

Pharmacologic management of cardiovascular disease includes antiplatelet agents, beta-blockers, angiotensin-converting enzyme (ACE) inhibitors, angiotensin receptor blockers (ARBs), statins, and diuretics.[5,8] Antiplatelet therapy, including aspirin and P2Y12 receptor inhibitors, such as clopidogrel, prasugrel, and ticagrelor, is an essential component of the management of cardiovascular disease. These agents inhibit platelet activation and aggregation, reducing the risk of thrombotic events, such as myocardial infarction and stroke.[10] In patients with acute coronary syndrome, dual antiplatelet therapy (DAPT) with aspirin and a P2Y12 receptor inhibitor is the standard of care. This regimen is also used in patients undergoing PCI to reduce the risk of stent thrombosis. However, the optimal duration of DAPT in these patients is a topic of ongoing research, with recent studies suggesting that shorter durations of therapy may be as effective as longer durations.[8,10] Studies indicate women have increased platelet reactivity compared with men.[10] The contributing factors for this sex difference are not definitively identified. It is postulated that higher levels of estrogen in women, leading to increased platelet to platelet aggregation, increased platelet adhesion to fibrinogen, and platelet interaction with leukocytes may be contributing factors.[10]

ACE inhibitors and beta-blockers have different advantages. ACE inhibitors are particularly effective in reducing blood pressure and preventing cardiovascular events, such as stroke and heart attack.[2,8,10] They are also beneficial for patients with HF, as they improve cardiac function and reduce the risk for hospitalization.[8] ACE inhibitors are commonly used to treat hypertension and HF. ACE inhibitors work by blocking the enzyme that converts angiotensin I to angiotensin II. This results in the dilation of blood vessels and a decrease in blood pressure, reducing the workload on the heart.[11] ACE inhibitors have been shown to reduce the risk of stroke, heart attack, and other cardiovascular events. ACE inhibitors and beta-blockers have different advantages. Beta-blockers are commonly used to treat hypertension, HF, and angina. Beta-blockers work by blocking the effects of adrenaline and noradrenaline, reducing heart rate and blood pressure, and improving blood flow to the heart. Beta-blockers have been shown to reduce the risk of heart attack, arrhythmias, and sudden death.[2,5] Beta-blockers are particularly effective in reducing the risk of sudden death in patients with heart disease.

They also improve symptoms of angina, such as chest pain and shortness of breath, and reduce the risk of arrhythmias. Beta-blockers are also used to treat hypertension and HF and can improve exercise tolerance in patients with heart disease. Beta-blockers reduce mortality in patients with HF, whereas ACE inhibitors and ARBs decrease morbidity and mortality in patients with left ventricular dysfunction.[5,8]

Statin therapy is recommended for prevention and management of CVD based on the results of randomized controlled trials and meta-analyses.[2,12] Statins reduce low-density lipoprotein (LDL) cholesterol levels and inflammation, lowering the risk of major cardiovascular events. Benefits of statins are proportional to the intensity of LDL cholesterol reduction, and the guidelines recommend achieving LDL cholesterol levels below 70 mg/dL in high-risk patients.[5,8,13] There are some limitations to the evidence on statin therapy. Most studies on statins have enrolled male populations, with limited representation of women. Second, the benefits of statins may be offset by adverse effects, such as myalgia, hepatic dysfunction, and increased risk of diabetes. Third, the optimal duration and intensity of statin therapy are not well-defined, and the guidelines have undergone several revisions over time.[13]

Meta-analysis noted that statin therapy reduced the risk of major cardiovascular events by 20% in women, which aligned with the reduction observed in men.[12,13] However, the absolute risk reduction was smaller in women than in men, because of the lower baseline risk of CVD in women. Statin therapy did not reduce the risk of stroke or all-cause mortality in women.[12] Statins reduce LDL cholesterol and decrease the risk of cardiovascular events in both men and women; however, more women report not being offered statins in the prevention or management of CVD.[12,14–16]

Diuretics are useful in the acute and chronic management of fluid overload in patients with HF.[5,8] Diuretic therapy can help reduce fluid buildup in the body, leading to a decrease in symptoms and improved quality of life for patients with HF.[12] Although diuretic therapy can be effective in managing CVD, it is not without potential side effects.[5] Common side effects of diuretics include electrolyte imbalances, dehydration, and hypotension. These side effects should be managed through careful monitoring of patients' fluid and electrolyte balance and adjusting medication dosages as needed.[5,12,16]

### Complications/Concerns

CVD can significantly impact physical and emotional quality of life. Patients with CVD may experience fatigue, shortness of breath, chest pain, and difficulty performing activities of daily living. These symptoms can limit patients' ability to work, exercise, enjoy intimacy, and engage in other activities, leading to a reduced quality of life.[7,9,13] The overall effect of CVD on quality of life should be consistently evaluated by health care providers to gain insight into the daily lived experience of patients.[7,9] Ability to accomplish activities of daily living, signs of depression, and effect on interpersonal relationships should be components of the evaluation.[9,17]

CVD is a major risk factor for erectile dysfunction (ED), which can affect quality of life and intimacy.[18–20] The pathophysiology of ED in men with CVD is complex and multifactorial. Several factors contribute to the development of ED in men, including endothelial dysfunction, neurogenic dysfunction, and pharmacologic therapy for CVD.[21] Endothelial dysfunction is a common underlying mechanism of both CVD and ED, with impaired endothelial function resulting in reduced nitric oxide (NO) production and impaired vasodilation.[21] Arterial stiffness also contributes to reduced blood flow to the penis. Neurogenic dysfunction owing to CVD, including autonomic dysfunction and peripheral neuropathy, results in impaired neural signaling to the penis.[21] Medications used to manage symptoms of CVD (eg, antihypertensives, lipid-lowering drugs, thiazide-type diuretics, beta-blockers, selective serotonin reuptake inhibitors, cimetidine, and spironolactone) can lead to changes in vascular structures in the penis, contributing to ED.[17]

Erectile function can be assessed using validated questionnaires, such as the International Index of Erectile Function or the Sexual Health Inventory for Men. These questionnaires can help to identify the severity of ED and monitor treatment response.[20] Treatment is usually initiated with phosphodiesterase type 5 inhibitors, such as sildenafil, tadalafil, and vardenafil. These medications improve erectile function by enhancing the effects of NO, which increases penile blood flow.[21] The management of ED in men receiving medical treatment for CVD requires a multidisciplinary approach, involving collaboration between cardiologists, urologists, and primary health care providers.[19,20] The primary goal of treatment is to improve erectile function while minimizing the risk of adverse cardiovascular events.[21]

### Considerations

Sexual satisfaction is a contributing, but often overlooked, quality-of-life indicator.[17,20] In addition, sexual dysfunction is not limited to male gender. Women also experience levels of sexual dysfunction and dissatisfaction, although data are limited. Although men may report more frequent sexual problems, women experience more severe functional issues, including vaginal atrophy.[22] In women, vasocongestion and vaginal lubrication require effective vascular dilation and adequate blood supply. CVD and subsequent pharmacologic management can directly impact vaginal vasocongestion and lubrication, decreasing sexual satisfaction in women.[17,20,22] Women's sexual satisfaction may be evaluated via standard, validated screening tools, such as Larsen's Sexual Satisfaction Questionnaire and the Female Sexual Function Index. National advisory groups recommend routine clinical assessment of sexual problems and delivery of sexual counseling with all patients experiencing CVD.[22]

Transgender individuals face unique health challenges, including CVD. Transgender individuals are at a higher risk of developing CVD owing to several factors. Studies have shown that hormone replacement therapy (HRT) can lead to an increased risk of blood clots, hypertension, and heart disease. Transgender women who take estrogen and progesterone may be at a higher risk for clotting disorders and venous thromboembolism.[23,24] The transgender community is growing, which necessitates additional research on CVD risks and management, which is inclusive of this vulnerable population. Health care providers must work to provide risk reduction and comprehensive care of CVD in all populations.[23]

One of the primary ways to mitigate the risks of CVD in transgender individuals is to move beyond the basic provision of comprehensive hormone therapy management (HRT). Close monitoring of hormone levels and therapeutic medication administration management are also necessary to prevent poor health outcomes.[23] Patients undergoing HRT should receive regular check-ups, including cholesterol and blood pressure monitoring, to identify and address any potential issues. Health care providers must educate their patients on the potential side effects of hormone therapy and the importance of adhering to the prescribed dose to prevent any adverse effects.[24] Transgender individuals may experience discrimination and stigma, leading to social isolation, stress, and a higher prevalence of depression, which are all known risk factors for CVD.[23] Transgender individuals must be treated with dignity and respect. Health care providers must be trained in how to provide care that is inclusive and sensitive to the needs of all individuals and genders.[24]

Social determinants of health (SDH) also contribute to the development of CVD.[3,6] The SDH of CVD can be broadly categorized into the following domains:

- Social and economic environment: Poverty, unemployment, low socioeconomic status (SES), and social exclusion are associated with a higher risk of CVD. These factors are linked to limited access to healthy food, safe and affordable housing, and education, which can lead to unhealthy lifestyles and chronic stress.[25]
- Physical environment: The built environment, such as housing, transportation, and access to recreational spaces, can impact physical activity levels and access to healthy food. Exposure to environmental pollutants, such as air pollution, can also increase the risk of CVD.[26]
- Health behaviors: Lifestyle factors, such as smoking, physical inactivity, unhealthy diet, and excessive alcohol consumption, are major contributors to CVD.[7,9] These behaviors are often influenced by cultural norms, social support, and personal beliefs.[25,27,28]
- Health care access and quality: Access to health care services and the quality of care can impact the prevention, detection, and management of CVD. This includes access to preventive services, affordable medications, and cardiac rehabilitation programs.[7,26]

Addressing the SDH of CVD requires a comprehensive approach that includes both upstream policy interventions and downstream individual-level interventions.[24,27] One of the significant factors is SES. People with lower SES have a higher risk of CVD than those with higher SES. This is because of cumulative social risk, including racial minority, single living, low income, and low educational status, in addition to a lack of access to healthy food, health care, education, and safe environments within impoverished communities.[27] In addition, lower SES individuals are more likely to experience chronic stress, which is linked to the development of CVD.[6,7] Certain ethnic groups, such as African Americans and Hispanics, have a higher incidence of diseases such as hypertension and type II diabetes, which contribute to the development of CVD.[2,28] Contributing factors include lack of access to health care services, low SES, and cultural beliefs that contribute to unhealthy behaviors.[28,29]

Targeting the SDH that contributes to CVD may provide a strategy for risk reduction. One strategy is to improve access to healthy food sources by increasing the availability of fresh fruits and vegetables in low-income areas.[25] Supporting access to physical activity facilities or safe walking paths can provide opportunities for exercise and stress reduction.[25] Another strategy is to improve access to health care. This can be achieved by expanding health care coverage and targeted recruitment of health care providers into underserved areas. In addition, health care providers should be trained to provide culturally appropriate care to patients from different ethnic groups.[25,26] Stress reduction can be encouraged by incorporating stress reduction techniques, such as yoga, meditation, and deep breathing. Increasing access to mental health providers to promote stress reduction and management techniques may be beneficial.[26,28] Considering measures of social context with clear predictive value is feasible and affordable to collect on patients in clinical settings to inform medical decision making.[28] Efforts to promote the change in basic assumptions focusing solely on disease treatment must be expanded to include health promotion for all people owing to the strong potential for positive impact on improved quality of life and health outcomes.

## SUMMARY

CVD is a significant public health issue affecting both men and women, but gender-specific differences in manifestation, risk factors, and outcomes must be considered when managing the disease. Implementing gender-specific management strategies, such as risk factor stratification and modification, diagnosis and treatment, increased access to cardiac rehabilitation, and expanded access to care, can improve outcomes and reduce gender disparities. Targeted approaches to improve quality of life for patients with CVD should be a priority for health care providers. Focusing on prevention and early intervention strategies through education on lifestyle modification, healthy diet, routine activity, and smoking cessation should be standard components of each wellness visit. Routine screening for cholesterol, hypertension, and familial risk factors may identify patients in need of additional evaluation. Increased access to health care, including preventative care, early intervention, and effective treatment options, is essential to improve health outcomes. Increasing access also includes affordable medications, procedures, therapies, and health care providers.

Gender and gender identity require consideration in the management of CVD owing to the different effects based on gender and gender identity. CVD affects women differently than men. Studies have demonstrated women are more likely to experience atypical symptoms of CAD and CVD, which can create diagnostic challenges. Women are also more likely to experience complications from CVD, such as HF, arrhythmias, and stroke, compared with men. These gender-based differences must be considered when developing treatment plans and managing CVD in women. Transgender individuals may face additional risk factors. Transgender individuals, particularly those undergoing hormone therapy, may face increased risk of developing hypertension and insulin resistance. Health care providers must be aware of these risk factors and take them into account when managing CVD in transgender patients. Gender-affirming care is crucial to health outcomes and well-being. Gender-affirming care refers to health care that recognizes and affirms a patient's gender identity. For transgender individuals with CVD, gender-affirming care includes using a patient's preferred name and pronouns, providing access to gender-affirming hormone therapy, and considering the unique health needs of transgender individuals. Addressing bias and discrimination in health care settings is necessary to improve the quality of care all individuals receive. Health care providers must work collectively and collaboratively to address and eliminate any biases or discrimination that may exist in their practice.

Health care providers must also consider gender-related pharmacokinetic and pharmacodynamic differences in response to medications. Women may require lower doses of certain medications because of their smaller body size, lower levels of certain enzymes, and effects of sex hormones before and after menopause. Women may also have a higher risk of adverse drug reactions because of hormonal differences, genetic variations, and drug interactions. Discounting the impact of gender differences in response to medications can result in suboptimal treatment and adverse outcomes. It is therefore essential to consider gender as a critical factor when developing treatment plans for patients with CVD.

Further research is needed to identify and understand the gender differences in CVD to develop effective gender-specific management strategies. Clinical trial results are used to guide practice, and it is important that these results can be applied within diverse patient populations. It is important to ensure that women have equal access to the benefits of medical research and are not unnecessarily denied opportunities. By excluding women from clinical trials, researchers may be eliminating discovery of new, effective treatment options.[28,29] Through inclusive clinical trials, researchers can ensure that the results are generalizable to both sexes and that treatments are effective for all patients. Recognizing gender-specific differences in the prevalence, pathophysiology, diagnosis, and management of CVD is essential for promoting optimal health outcomes. Clinicians should be aware of gender-related differences and tailor approaches to reduce risks and improve outcomes, including quality of life, for all patients with CVD.

## CLINICS CARE POINTS

- Screening and Diagnosis: Women are less likely to be screened for cardiovascular disease than men. Women may have atypical symptoms that are often dismissed or misdiagnosed.[2–4] Health care providers should be aware of these gender-specific differences and ensure that women are screened and diagnosed appropriately.[2–4] This may involve using different diagnostic tests or criteria for women, as well as considering gender-specific risk factors.[3]

- Lifestyle Modifications: Lifestyle modifications, such as diet and exercise, are important components of the management of cardiovascular disease in both men and women. However, there may be gender-specific differences in the effectiveness of these interventions. For example, women may require different exercise regimens or dietary modifications than men and may also benefit from targeted interventions to address their unique risk factors, such as menopause or pregnancy-related complications.[5–7,9]

- Risk factor modification: Both men and women should be encouraged to adopt a healthy lifestyle and manage their cardiovascular risk factors. However, women may require more aggressive risk factor management owing to their higher prevalence of comorbidities and unique risk factors, such as gestational hypertension, preeclampsia, and menopause.[5,6,11]

- Diagnosis and treatment: Women are often misdiagnosed or undertreated for cardiovascular disease owing to atypical symptoms and underrepresentation in clinical trials. Therefore, health care providers should be educated on the gender differences in cardiovascular disease presentation and treatment and should consider using gender-specific diagnostic tools and treatment algorithms.[2,3,6]

- Treatment: Although the overall treatment goals for cardiovascular disease are the same for men and women, there may be gender-specific differences in the optimal treatment approach. For example, women may respond differently to certain medications or interventions and may require different dosages or durations of treatment. Women are also more likely to experience adverse effects from some medications, such as aspirin and statins, which may require adjustments in the treatment plan.[12–15]

- Cardiac rehabilitation: Both men and women should be offered cardiac rehabilitation after a cardiac event or procedure, as it has been shown to improve outcomes and quality of life. However, women may require tailored rehabilitation programs that address their unique needs, such as addressing menopausal symptoms, managing comorbidities, and reducing caregiver burden.[2,3]

- Patient Education and Support: Women may face unique challenges in managing their cardiovascular disease, such as balancing their caregiving responsibilities with their own health needs.[7,22,23] Health care providers should provide education and support that is tailored to the specific needs and experiences of women, including addressing any barriers to adherence to treatment and providing resources for managing stress and mental health.[12,23,24]

- Policy interventions: Policies that address the social and economic determinants of cardiovascular disease, such as poverty reduction, income redistribution, and investment in education and housing, can improve health outcomes.[27,28] Environmental policies that promote active transportation, clean air, and access to healthy food can also reduce the risk of cardiovascular disease.[27,28]

- Community-based interventions: Community-based interventions that promote healthy lifestyles, such as physical activity and healthy eating, can improve cardiovascular health. These interventions should be tailored to the specific needs of the community and address social and cultural factors that influence health behaviors.[28,29]

- Health system interventions: Health system interventions, such as improving access to preventive services, medications, and cardiac rehabilitation, can improve the detection and management of cardiovascular disease. These interventions should address barriers to access, such as cost, transportation, communication, and health literacy.[25,26,29]

**DISCLOSURE**

The authors declare no conflict of interest.

**REFERENCES**

1. World Health Organization. Cardiovascular Diseases. Available at: https://www.who.int/health-topics/cardiovascular-diseases#tab=tab_1. Accessed February 16, 2023.
2. Humphries KH, Lee MK, Izadnegahdar M, et al. Sex differences in cardiovascular disease – impact on care and outcomes. Front Neuroendocrinol 2017;46:46–70.
3. Biddle C, Fallavollita JA, Homish GG, et al. Gender differences in symptom misattribution for coronary heart disease symptoms and intentions to seek health care. Womens Health 2019;60(4):367–81.
4. Mackey C, Diercks DB. Gender bias in the management of patients still exists. Acad Emerg Med 2018;25(4):467–9.
5. De Bellis A, Angelis G, Fabris E, et al. Gender-related differences in heart failure: beyond the 'one-size-fits-all' paradigm. Heart Fail Rev 2019;25(2):245–55.
6. Kalman MB, Wells M, Fahs PS, et al. Educating rural women about gender specific heart attack and prodromal symptoms. Online J Rural Nurs Health Care 2018;18(2):113–33.
7. Darma A, Bertagnolli L, Torri F, et al. Gender differences in patients with structural heart disease undergoing VT ablation. J Cardiovasc Electrophysiol 2021;32(10):2675–83.
8. Myerson RM, Colantonio LD, Safford MM, et al. Does identification of previously undiagnosed conditions change care-seeking behavior? Health Serv Res 2018;53(3):1517–38.
9. Kong D, Lu P, Solomon P, et al. Gender-based depression trajectories following heart disease onset: significant predictors and health outcomes. Aging Ment Health 2021;26(4):754–61.
10. Schreuder MM, Bidal R, Boersma E, et al. Efficacy and safety of high potent P2Y inhibitors prasugrel and ticagrelor in patients with coronary heart disease treated with dual antiplatelet therapy: a sex-specific systematic review and meta-analysis. J Am Heart Assoc 2020;9(4). https://doi.org/10.1161/jaha.119.014457.
11. Herman LL, Padala SA, Ahmed I, et al. Angiotensin converting enzyme inhibitors (ACEI) [Updated 2022 Aug 5]. In: StatPearls [Internet]. Treasure Island (FL): StatPearls Publishing; 2022 Jan-. Available at: https://www.ncbi.nlm.nih.gov/books/NBK431051/. Accessed February 18, 2023.
12. Wall HK, Ritchey MD, Gillespi C, et al. Vital signs: prevalence of key cardiovascular disease risk factors for million hearts 2022 - United States, 2011-2016. MMWR (Morb Mortal Wkly Rep): Morb Mortal Wkly Rep 2018;67(35):983–91.
13. Buchanan CH, Brown EA, Bishu KG, et al. The magnitude and potential causes of sex disparities in statin therapy in veterans with type 2 diabetes: a 10-year nationwide longitudinal cohort study. Womens Health Issues 2022;32(3):274–83.
14. Nanna MG, Wang TY, Xian Q, et al. Sex differences in the use of statins in community practice. Circulation: Cardiovascular Quality & Outcomes 2019;12(8):1–10.
15. Carr L. Aspirin and statin prescription for CVD prevention. Contemp Ob Gyn 2021;66(11):25.
16. Heo S, Shin MS, Hwang SY, et al. Sex differences in heart failure symptoms and factors associated with heart failure symptoms. J Cardiovasc Nurs 2019;34(4):306–12.

17. Gök F, Demir Korkmaz F. Sexual counseling provided by cardiovascular nurses: attitudes, beliefs, perceived barriers, and proposed solutions. J Cardiovasc Nurs 2018;33(6):E24–30.
18. Sex hormones and your heart. Harv Womens Health Watch 2019;26(9):1–7.
19. Long M, Fink R. Erectile dysfunction: harbinger of early cardiovascular disease. Clinical Advisor 2021;24(2):12–20.
20. East L, Jackson D, Manias E, et al. Patient perspectives and experiences of sexual health conversations and cardiovascular disease: a qualitative study. J Clin Nurs 2021;30(21/22):3194–204.
21. Andersson K-E, Andersson KE. PDE5 inhibitors - pharmacology and clinical applications 20 years after sildenafil discovery. Br J Pharmacol 2018;175(13):2554–65.
22. Smith AB, Barton DL. Prevalence and severity of sexual dysfunction and sexual dissatisfaction in coronary artery disease: an integrative review. Can J Cardiovasc Nurs 2020;30(2):22–30.
23. Poteat TC, Shahrzad D, Streed CG Jr, et al. Cardiovascular disease in a population-based sample of transgender and cisgender adults. Am J Prev Med 2021;61(6):804–11.
24. Knight EP. Gender and cardiovascular disease risk: beyond the binary. J Nurse Pract 2021;17(7):823–7.
25. Al Rifai M, Jia X, Pickett J, et al. Social determinants of health and comorbidities among individuals with atherosclerotic cardiovascular disease: the behavioral risk factor surveillance system survey. Popul Health Manag 2022;25(1):39–45.
26. Mannoh I, Hussein M, Commodore-Mensah Y, et al. Impact of social determinants of health on cardiovascular disease prevention. Curr Opin Cardiol 2021;36(5):572–9.
27. Canterbury Ann, Echouffo-Tcheugui JB, Shpilsky D, et al. Association between cumulative social risk, particulate matter environmental pollutant exposure, and cardiovascular disease risk. BMC Cardiovasc Disord 2020;20(1):1–7.
28. Hamad R, Glymour MM, Calmasini C, et al. Explaining the variance in cardiovascular disease risk factors: a comparison of demographic, socioeconomic, and genetic predictors. Epidemiology 2022;33(1):25–33.
29. Lloyd-Jones DM, Allen NB, Anderson CAM, et al. Life's essential 8: updating and enhancing the American heart association's construct of cardiovascular health: a presidential advisory from the American heart association. Circulation 2022;146:e18–43.

# Hospice and Palliative Care– Men and Gender-Specific Roles

Brent MacWilliams, PhD, APNP, ANP-BC[a],*, Erin McArthur, MLIS[b]

## KEYWORDS

- Palliative care • Palliative care specialties • Hospice care • End of life • Gender
- Gender role • Gender equity • Gender norms

## KEY POINTS

- Gender is not reflected in the binary definition of male and female and should be viewed as a complex construct.
- Gender norms and inequalities affect health outcomes for men and gender minorities in palliative care and hospice care.
- Clinicians in all specialties need to be aware of best practices related to palliative and hospice care and competent to access those services.
- Alzheimer/dementia/Parkinson, cancer/oncology, and heart failure diagnoses all have highly evolved specialized palliative care services, evidence-based guidelines, and significant research to guide practice.
- Men and gender minorities have specialized issues that need to be assessed and addressed to provided optimal care.

## INTRODUCTION

All people face end of life as the final health outcome, and as people age or face major health status changes, the health priorities change. When a person's health focus shifts from quantity to quality of life, palliative care (PC) comes into view. When a person's health status changes so significantly or deteriorates to the point that end-of-life appears to be imminent (approximately 6 months), then hospice comes into view. Clinicians serving patients across the health care spectrum must be aware of the nature and efficacy of palliative and hospice care (HC), indications for referral to services, and current best practices. Creating an end-of-life trajectory requires an individualized and global personal plan, which PC and HC can provide. Gender-specific care that includes gender minorities provides special and unique challenges to those seeking PC and HC.

[a] University of Wisconsin-Oshkosh, College of Nursing, 800 Algoma Boulevard, Oshkosh, WI 54901, USA; [b] University of Wisconsin-Oshkosh Libraries
* Corresponding author.
*E-mail address:* macwillb@uwosh.edu

Nurs Clin N Am 58 (2023) 607–615
https://doi.org/10.1016/j.cnur.2023.06.004
0029-6465/23/© 2023 Elsevier Inc. All rights reserved.

nursing.theclinics.com

## GENDER REIMAGED

Gender (in contrast to biologic sex) refers to culturally defined roles and attributes associated with being or appearing to be a woman or a man; the gender binary refers to a system of considering and categorizing gender in which all people are either male or female.[1-3] Although many people experience their gender identity as falling within these categories of man or woman, others do not. In the 1990's, the term genderqueer emerged to describe someone who felt their gender lay outside of the binary, between male and female, or not completely identifying with one specific binary identity.[4] Genderqueer may be used as an umbrella term for any gender outside of male and female, or may have a uniquely rebellious connotation as a challenge to the master gender binary narrative.[4] Nonbinary began to appear in the lexicon shortly after genderqueer, and the broader and more inclusive term gender diverse is an even more recent term. Gender diverse has been defined as a term that "recognizes and celebrates that all people express a gender identity, and that gender identity and expression are not necessarily linked to a person's sex."[5] Clinicians may be more familiar with the term transgender, which describes people whose internal knowledge of their own gender does not align with the sex they were assigned at birth.[6,7] However, some nonbinary people do not identify as transgender, and consequently may face discrimination from both outside and inside the transgender community.[8] Although nonbinary people have always existed, research around nonbinary identities is new and limited; as most research focuses on the transgender population, most clinicians have not been offered education on how to work with nonbinary people.[8]

## GENDER AS A HEALTH CARE CONSTRUCT

The gender binary is a highly patriarchal system, assigning "greater value to men and things considered to be masculine than to women or things considered to be feminine," and "grant[ing] less legitimacy to gender identities or expressions that do not conform"[1(p2441)]. Gender norms are the glue holding this system together. Gender norms can be defined as "social norms defining acceptable and appropriate actions for women and men in a given group or society. They are embedded in formal and informal institutions, nested in the mind, and produced and reproduced through social interaction"[9(p415-6)]. Restrictive gender norms and the pervasiveness of the gender binary have a significant impact on health outcomes, both for individuals who identify within the gender binary and those who do not. Health systems reinforce gender norms, resulting in poorer outcomes for women, men, and gender minorities. Gender norms dictate men's and women's domains (eg, services for women are often focused on their reproductive and caregiving capacity, while at the same time, clinicians often resist men's engagement in maternal and pediatric care).[10] Although women have higher risks than men for certain conditions, including depression, anxiety, cancer, and aging-related health burdens, they may receive worse care; stereotypes of women as fragile and emotional can lead to their health complaints being perceived as exaggerated or being attributed to psychosomatic causes.[1,11] Gender norms around masculinity can lead to clinicians viewing men as strong, not needing care, and less compliant than female patients, despite men's lower life expectancy and many higher health risks relative to women.[11] Gender biases can be exacerbated when clinicians encounter patients who represent a gender or sexual minority. Nonbinary individuals face unique barriers in health care, many of which are not experienced by transgender people. Nonbinary people may experience worse mental health outcomes and higher rates of suicide than their binary transgender peers.[12] Gendered language and policies in health care settings, such as "reassigning" nonbinary patients within a binary gender, can create barriers, resulting in a breakdown of trust and unwillingness to seek needed care.[13] Consequently, nonbinary people and other gender minorities are more likely to delay care, putting them at risk for chronic health issues. Nonbinary people may have difficulty accessing gender-affirming medical or surgical care if providers do not consider them to be truly transgender, as the dominant medical narrative requires a transition from 1 binary gender to another.[8,12]

## GENDER-SPECIFIC DISCUSSIONS/IMPLICATIONS

In hospice care (HC) and palliative care (PC), gender norms and expectations can be an obstacle to universally beneficial care. Inside the gender binary, gender norms fail both men and women, as ingrained beliefs dictate group expectations and how health care providers treat them.[14–16] In an ethnographic study of the context and culture of palliative care, participants who had practiced traditional gender roles before illness found those roles deepening and in 1 case, becoming "symbolic of life itself" ([p31]). Changes in these entrenched gender roles at the end of life can be distressing; the gendered expectation that men should be independent can cause men to experience depression at the end of life, when they become dependent on their caregivers.[15] The impact of gender norms goes beyond patients' internalized beliefs; in their scoping review on gender disparities in end-of-life care,[15] researchers found that deeply ingrained gender bias permeated multiple domains, including caregiving, symptom experience, care preferences, and coping strategies. For example, health care providers were more likely to delegate physical care tasks to women, who were assumed to be inherently more compassionate and willing to put others before themselves; providers offered more support to male caregivers, who were perceived as heroic for providing care outside of their traditional gender role.[15,17] Researchers found that "male patients mainly rely on social support from partners, have higher expectations to be cared for at home, and have higher need for preservation of autonomy" ([p8]). For nonbinary and gender diverse people, the pervasiveness of the gender binary in HC and PC can cause significant distress. Patients may fear that their providers will misgender them or use incorrect names or pronouns, or that they will be forced to use gender-specific bathrooms or shared bedrooms.[18] Barriers to PC are also under the global influence of ethnocultural norms, which have a broad influence that engulfs gender.[19] Gender minorities include men, so both binary and nonbinary research studies are combined in the literature review for this work. Regardless of gender orientation, people all share the same health care trajectory but may have different experiences when accessing and receiving PC and HC.

## PALLIATIVE CARE TO HOSPICE CARE TRAJECTORY
### Palliative Care Overview

PC focuses on "expert assessment and management of pain and other symptoms, assessment and support of caregiver needs, and coordination of care."[20] PC uses a team-based approach to meet the physical, psychological, and adaptive changes needed, and spiritual consequences of a serious illness. PC is a person-centric and family-centered approach to providing people who are seriously ill with relief from the global illness effects. PC is not the end of curative or life-prolonging interventions but a supportive service that can be provided in tandem with the current health care team. PC is provided based on the patient's need for increased support, including management of symptoms, support of caregiver needs, and coordination of care. PC is based on patient needs and not the patient's prognosis.[20–22] PC is provided by health systems, independent provider practices, cancer centers, dialysis units, home health agencies, hospices, and long-term care providers. Professional services are provided by a diverse interdisciplinary team, based on the patient's needs and the PC setting. The PC team would typically include nurse practitioners, doctors, nurses, and social workers, but could also include chaplains, counselors, pharmacists, dietitians, rehabilitation specialists, physical therapists, music and art therapists, and home health aides. The PC team assesses the needs and desires of the patient, identified family members, and caregiver(s) in coordination with the current health care team.[21–26]

### Hospice Care Overview

HC is relatively new compared with other health care specialty practices. In 1979, the Health Care Financing Administration (HCFA) initiated demonstration programs at 26 hospices in 16 states to assess the cost-effectiveness of HC and to help determine what a hospice is and what it should provide and new standards and guidelines were established.[27] Hospice is defined as "the model for quality, compassionate care for people facing a life-limiting illness or injury, hospice care involves a team-oriented approach to expert medical care, pain management, and emotional and spiritual support expressly tailored to the patient's needs and wishes."[28] "Hospice focuses on caring, not curing" and care is provided in the most supportive setting, which is often in the patient's home.[29] In 1982, Congress created a Medicare provision, so HC became a Medicare benefit. Today, everyone 65 years and older who enrolled in Medicare can access HC as a benefit. In 2020, $22.4 billion were spent on HC, and 1.72 million Medicare beneficiaries were enrolled in HC for 1 day or more.[29] Hospice services are available to patients of any age, religion, race, or illness and covered under Medicaid, most private insurance plans, health maintenance organizations (HMOs), and other managed care organizations. An HC referral should be explored by clinicians when end of life is expected in less than 6 months, especially when there is almost unlimited access to the services.[22,29]

### Care Setting and Population

HC and PC are extensions on the same continuum or trajectory. PC services like HC services have become part of the fabric of the health care system. "Since 2000, the percentage of hospitals (with 50 or more beds) with a palliative care program has more than tripled. As of 2020, more than 83% of these hospitals had a palliative care team."[21] Specialized PC services to serve patients with rapidly changing health status expanded during the pandemic years with the goal of improving quality, which has also reduced cost.[21,22] Increasing the referral network to community-based palliative care programs (home, assisted living facility, and long-term care) must be the focus for the PC growth phase moving forward.[21] HC services are similar PC and provided in hospitals, freestanding hospice centers, nursing homes and other long-term care facilities.[28] In the HC Medicare hospice beneficiary's population, Alzheimer/dementias/Parkinson remained the largest population by primary diagnoses (18.5%), followed by heart failure/circulatory (9.3%) and cancer diagnosis (7.5%).[29] The patient populations accessing PC care is more diverse but similar by diagnosis to the HC population. According to the National Hospice and Palliative Care Organization (NHPCO) Palliative Care Needs Survey, the top 6 requested service needs in PC are: symptom management, patient/family education, goals of care discussions, advance care planning, comprehensive assessment, and care coordination. The survey reflects the growing need for PC services as part of an emerging and expanding health care specialty.

### Discussion/Implications

Alzheimer/dementia/Parkinson, cancer/oncology, and heart failure diagnoses all have highly evolved specialized PC services, evidence-based guidelines, and significant research to guide practice.[20,30–34]

Patients diagnosed with any of the dementias face no definitive cure and a longer more insidious trajectory. Early diagnosis provides time for patients and their family to move through the grieving process, providing time for advanced care planning. Survival is variable, and reported means or medians range between 3 and 10 years [33,35] Health care professionals dealing with dementia patients need specific expertise in communication with patients who have cognitive impairment and their families, managing behavioral problems, anticipating, assessing, and managing physical problems.[24,25,33] Patients diagnosed with dementia have the highest HC use in the Medicare population.[29] Martinsson et al[36] in a 3-year study, researchers identified the importance of advance care planning and individual assessments in nursing homes to avoid referral to hospitals. The researchers also found that younger age and male gender patients with advanced dementia who died in the hospital setting were associated with poorer quality of end-of-life care compared to death in nursing homes.[37] Researchers found that people with advanced dementia have complex health care needs and benefit from PC interventions and integration of PC, early in the course of the disease. They also found that common causes of death for people with dementia include pneumonia, cardiovascular disease, and sudden, unexplained deaths. Further, they found the women's postdiagnosis survival time (4.1–4.3 years) was significantly longer than for men (4.6–5.1 years).[37] The quality of life for the late-stage dementia patient in assisted living facilities that specialize in that type of care appears to be optimal (Steen and colleagues, 2014).[33]

Sobanski et al,[32] identified early introduction and integration of palliative care in patients with heart failure improves quality of life. "Men prone to macrovascular coronary artery disease and myocardial infarction are at almost twice the risk of HF with reduced ejection fraction (HFrEF) and are usually younger at the time they are affected by HF than women."[32] According to Higashitsuji and colleagues,[38] advance care planning (APC) for heart failure patients resulted in improving quality of life and patient satisfaction while reducing readmissions among patients and reduced overall medical costs. A Delphi study looking at criteria for referral of patients with advanced heart failure for specialized palliative care "reached consensus on a large number of criteria for referral to specialist palliative care and concluded that with further validation, these criteria may be useful for standardizing palliative care access in the inpatient and/or outpatient settings."[39]

Cancer patients may experience a substantial decline in function in the last months or weeks of life, and diseased trajectories are relatively well-defined.[40] According to Cloyes and colleagues,[41] sexual and gender minority cancer survivors (after diagnosis to end of life) can face inadequate palliative services and end of life cancer care.[42] Researchers identified the barriers to LGBT PC in cancer were based on mistrust of health care providers coupled with a lack of health care provider LGBT-specific knowledge. The researchers identified significant downstream effects like discrimination, criminalization, persecution, fear, distress, social isolation, disenfranchised grief, bereavement, tacit acknowledgment, and homophobia.[43,44] Researchers found women and younger adult patients with advanced cancer require special attention and support because of symptom burden. Palliative care and supportive care (PSC) were combined as a care model that improved the quality of life for male patients with genitourinary malignancies and during their cancer journey[43,44] found males and younger patients who received early palliative care (EPC) had better quality of life and mood than those who received oncology care alone. The researchers also found that in advanced cancer care an improvement in quality of life for females assigned to PC but not for males; these findings differ from a prior randomized trial evaluating a multidisciplinary team intervention.[45] Overall, it appears that early PC intervention across the diagnostic spectrum results in a greater quality of life.[22,44,45]

### Indications for a Palliative Care/Hospice Referral

The greatest challenge and barrier identified by respondents to the NHPCO Palliative Care Needs Survey was "referring providers not understanding palliative care coupled with a lack of patients/families understanding of palliative care" (2020, p. 2). Regardless of the clinicians' practice setting, when a new serious illness or exacerbation of chronic illness changes the trajectory of a patient's health; it could be time for a PC and/or HC consultation. The PC team can help with managing complex pain, consult regarding the trajectory of comorbidities, and broker patient/family communication.[22,46] There are general referral criteria that have been developed to assess need for a PC consultation specific the practice setting.[22,46] There are evidence-based criteria for various other acute settings such as the intensive care unit (ICU), oncology, and the emergency department. If a patient meets one or more of the outlined criteria, then a referral to the palliative care team may be indicated.[46]

### Assessing Readiness

The referral process begins with a critical conversation (or series of conversations) to assess readiness. Clinicians are often hesitant to discuss palliative care and do not know the correct questions to ask and especially those that are more gender specific.[22] Asking permission to discuss the disease trajectory and what it means is a good place to start. Assessing the patients' understanding of their disease trajectory and those of identified family members to be gender inclusive is key. Be realistic but hopeful to frame a serious prognosis; if the conversation has progressed to the point of weighing options, then it is the perfect time for a PC or HC team consultation.[22,46]

### Challenges/Limitations

The emergence of gender as a nonbinary construct presents challenges and limitations for evidenced-based practice. The gender binary refers to a system of considering and categorizing gender in which all people are either male or female; this has been the excepted as the demographic standard in research but does not capture the emerging nonbinary construct, which makes capturing the entire population with divergent experiences difficult or impossible to capture without introducing gender bias in the findings. The body of current research is comprised of mixed binary and nonbinary data, which limits the applicability of even seminal historical work.

### FUTURE CONSIDERATIONS/SUMMARY

With the emerging social acceptance of a nonbinary gender construct, it is critical that health care providers become aware and trained to meet the needs of gender minorities; this will create a more inclusive practice environment for all patient regardless of their gender identify. When health care providers are open to change, self-aware, educated regarding gender issues, and ready to challenge assumptions, bias becomes less likely and patient care improves. The assessment, diagnostics, and treatment of all patients improve when patients are listened to, accepted for who they are and have inclusive plans tailored to their individual needs. Currently the health care experience for gender minorities is substandard care across the health care continuum, which includes PC and HC. The social pressure for men to meet the traditional vison of masculinity has its own set of limitations that can also result in less-than-optimal care. The key for clinicians is to be aware of gender as a social construct, become aware of their local PC and HC services, and become comfortable with making referrals.

## CLINICS CARE POINTS

- Gender is a fluid nonbinary continuium that should be assesed on a case by case basis.
- End of Life Care planning must be personal, individualized and inclusive.
- We are all on a terminal trajectory; so clinicians need to assess timing, and offer options so patients can make informed choices.
- Gender minorities often recieve substandard care due to bias and assumptions that apply to the majority populations.

## DISCLOSURE

The authors have nothing to disclose.

## REFERENCES

1. Heise L, Greene ME, Opper N, et al. Gender inequality and restrictive gender norms: framing the challenges to health. Lancet 2019;393(10189):2440–54.
2. Oxford University Press. (2023). Gender binary. In: Oxford learner's dictionaries. Available at: https://www.oxfordlearnersdictionaries.com/definition/english/gender-binary. Accessed February 07, 2023.
3. Saeed F, Hoerger M, Norton SA, et al. Preference for palliative care in cancer patients: are men and women alike? J Pain Symptom Manag 2018;56(1):1–6.e1.
4. Thorne N, Yip AK, Bouman WP, et al. The terminology of identities between, outside and beyond the gender binary - a systematic review. Int J Transgenderism 2019;20(2–3):138–54.
5. Winter S. Are human rights capable of liberation? The case of sex and gender diversity. Aust J Hum Right 2009;15(1):151–73.
6. GLAAD. (n.d.). Glossary of terms: transgender. Available at: https://www.glaad.org/reference/trans-terms. Accessed February 07, 2023.
7. Streed CG Jr. Health communication and sexual orientation, gender identity, and expression. Med Clin 2022;106(4):589–600.
8. National LGBT Health Education Center. (2016, November 15). Providing affirmative care for patients with non-binary gender identities. Available at: https://www.lgbtqiahealtheducation.org/publication/providing-affirmative-care-patients-non-binary-gender-identities/. Accessed February 20, 2023.
9. Cislaghi B, Heise L. Gender norms and social norms: Differences, similarities and why they matter in prevention science. Sociol Health Illness 2020;42(2):215–49.
10. Gupta GR, Oomman N, Grown C, et al, and Gender Equality, Norms, and Health Steering Committee. Gender equality and gender norms: framing the opportunities for health. Lancet 2019;393(10190):2550–62.
11. Hay K, McDougal L, Percival V, et al, Gender Equality, Norms, and Health Steering Committee. Disrupting gender norms in health systems: making the case for change. Lancet 2019;393(10190):2535–49.

12. Matsuno E, Budge SL. Non-binary/genderqueer identities: a critical review of the literature. Curr Sex Health Rep 2017;9:116–20.
13. Durocher K, Caxaj CS. Gender binaries in nursing: a critical shift to postgenderism. Nursing for Women's Health 2022;26(4):262–8.
14. Maingi S, Bagabag AE, O'Mahony S. Current best practices for sexual and gender minorities in hospice and palliative care settings. J Pain Symptom Manag 2018;55(5):1420–7.
15. Wong AD, Phillips SP. Gender disparities in end of life care: a scoping review. J Palliat Care 2023;38(1):78–96.
16. Hughes CR, Gremillion H. The meanings of gender and the home space for recipients of palliative care, and some implications for social workers in the field. Social Dialogue Magazine 2014;9:30–2.
17. Ullrich A, Grube K, Hlawatsch C, et al. Exploring the gender dimension of problems and needs of patients receiving specialist palliative care in a German palliative care unit - the perspectives of patients and healthcare professionals. BMC Palliat Care 2019;18(1). https://doi.org/10.1186/s12904-019-0440-7. Article 59.
18. Higgins A, Hynes G. Meeting the needs of people who identify as lesbian, gay, bisexual, transgender, and queer in palliative care settings. J Hospice Palliat Nurs 2019;21(4):286–90.
19. Busolo D, Woodgate R. Palliative care experiences of adult cancer patients from ethnocultural groups: A qualitative systematic review protocol. JBI Database of Systematic Reviews and Implementation Reports 2015;13(1):99–111.
20. Ferrell BR, Twaddle ML, Melnick A, et al. National Consensus Project clinical practice guidelines for quality palliative care guidelines, 4th edition. J Palliat Med 2018;21(12):1684–9.
21. Center to Advance Palliative Care (CAPC). (2022) Growth of palliative care in US hospitals: 2022 snapshot (2000 - 2020). Available at: https://www.capc.org/documents/download/1031/. Accessed February 20, 2023.
22. Tatum PE, Mills SS. Hospice and palliative care: an overview. Med Clin 2020; 104(3):359–73.
23. Myatra SN, Salins N, Iyer S, et al. End-of-life care policy: an integrated care plan for the dying: a joint position statement of the Indian Society of Critical Care Medicine (ISCCM) and the Indian Association of Palliative Care (IAPC). Indian J Crit Care Med 2014;18(9):615–35.
24. National Consensus Project for Quality Palliative Care. (2018). National Coalition for Hospice and Palliative Care Clinical Practice Guidelines for Quality Palliative Care. Definition of palliative care. Available at: NCHPC-NCPGuidelines_4thED_-web_FINAL. pdf (nationalcoalitionhpc. org). Accessed November 10, 2021.
25. National Hospice and Palliative Care Organization. (2020a). NHPCO facts and figures, 2020 edition. Available at: https://www.nhpco.org/wp-content/uploads/NHPCO-Facts-Figures-2020-edition.pdf. Accessed February 20, 2023.
26. National Hospice and Palliative Care Organization. (2020b). NHPCO palliative care needs survey. Available at: https://www.nhpco.org/2020-pc-needs-survey/. Accessed February 20, 2023.
27. National Hospice and Palliative Care Organization. (2023). History of hospice. Available at: https://www.nhpco.org/hospice-care-overview/history-of-hospice/. Accessed February 20, 2023.
28. National Hospice and Palliative Care Organization. (2023). Hospice care overview for professionals. Available at: https://www.nhpco.org/hospice-care-overview/. Accessed February 20, 2023.

29. National Hospice and Palliative Care Organization. (2022). NHPCO facts and figures, 2022 edition. Available at: https://www.nhpco.org/wp-content/uploads/NHPCO-Facts-Figures-2022.pdf. Accessed February 20, 2023.
30. Dans M, Kutner JS, Agarwal R, et al. NCCN Guidelines Insights: Palliative Care, Version 2.2021. J Natl Compr Cancer Netw 2021;19(7):780–8.
31. Hui D, Bruera E. Integrating palliative care into the trajectory of cancer care. Nat Rev Clin Oncol 2016;13(3):159–71.
32. Sobanski PZ, Krajnik M, Goodlin SJ. Palliative care for people living with heart disease - does sex make a difference? Frontiers in Cardiovascular Medicine 2021;8. https://doi.org/10.3389/fcvm.2021.629752. Article 629752.
33. van der Steen JT, Radbruch L, Hertogh CM, et al. White paper defining optimal palliative care in older people with dementia: a Delphi study and recommendations from the European Association for Palliative Care. Palliat Med 2014;28(3):197–209.
34. Visseren FLJ, Mach F, Smulders YM, et al, ESC Scientific Document Group. 2021 ESC Guidelines on cardiovascular disease prevention in clinical practice. Eur Heart J 2021;42(34):3227–337.
35. Tyrrell P, Harberger S, Schoo C, et al. Kubler-Ross stages of dying and subsequent models of grief. InStatPearls. StatPearls Publishing; 2022.
36. Martinsson L, Lundström S, Sundelöf J. Better quality of end-of-life care for persons with advanced dementia in nursing homes compared to hospitals: a Swedish national register study. BMC Palliat Care 2020;19(1). https://doi.org/10.1186/s12904-020-00639-5. Article 135.
37. Eisenmann Y, Golla H, Schmidt H, et al. Palliative care in advanced dementia. Front Psychiatr 2020;11. https://doi.org/10.3389/fpsyt.2020.00699. Article 699.
38. Higashitsuji A, Sano M, Majima T. Advance care planning experiences of patients with heart failure and their families: a qualitative systematic review protocol. JBI Evidence Synthesis 2023;21(2):441–8.
39. Chang YK, Allen LA, McClung JA, et al. Criteria for referral of patients with advanced heart failure for specialized palliative care. J Am Coll Cardiol 2022;80(4):332–44.
40. Cloyes KG, Candrian C. Palliative and end-of-life care for sexual and gender minority cancer survivors: a review of current research and recommendations. Curr Oncol Rep 2021;23(4). https://doi.org/10.1007/s11912-021-01034-w. Article 39.
41. Haviland K, Burrows Walters C, Newman S. Barriers to palliative care in sexual and gender minority patients with cancer: A scoping review of the literature. Health Soc Care Community 2021;29(2):305–18.
42. Galiano A, Schiavon S, Nardi M, et al. Simultaneous care in oncology: Assessment of benefit in relation to symptoms, sex, and age in 753 patients. Front Oncol 2022;12. https://doi.org/10.3389/fonc.2022.989713. Article 989713.
43. Saraiya B, Dale W, Singer EA, et al. Integration of palliative and supportive care into the management of genitourinary malignancies. American Society of Clinical Oncology Educational Book 2022;42:341–50.
44. Nipp RD, Greer JA, El-Jawahri A, et al. Age and gender moderate the impact of early palliative care in metastatic non-small cell lung cancer. Oncol 2016;21(1):119–26.
45. Lapid MI, Atherton PJ, Kung S, et al. Does gender influence outcomes from a multidisciplinary intervention for quality of life designed for patients with advanced cancer? Support Care Cancer 2013;21(9):2485–90.
46. Center to Advance Palliative Care (CAPC). (2023). For clinicians. Get palliative care. Available at: https://getpalliativecare.org/resources/clinicians. Accessed March 01, 2023.

# Men in Female-Dominated Nursing Specialties

Curry Joseph Bordelon, DNP, MBA, NNP-BC, CNE[a],*,
Jason Mott, PhD, RN[b], Erin McArthur, BA, MA[c],
Brent MacWilliams, PhD, APNP, ANP-BC[c,1]

## KEYWORDS

- Men in nursing • Male and nursing specialties • Men and nursing specialties
- Male nurses and NICU men • NICU

## KEY POINTS

- While numbers of men in the nursing profession have slowly increased, men in female-dominated specialty areas have not changed.
- Gender bias, discrimination, and bullying are reported among male nurses in certain specialty nursing environments.
- By diversifying the nursing workforce, there is a potential to enhance patient comfort, improve satisfaction, and promote a more inclusive, creative, and patient-focused health care environment.

## INTRODUCTION

The modern nursing profession has been around for more than 150 years. Starting with Nightingale, nursing took on a lead role in society. Over time, nursing has been viewed as the most caring profession. Many of the attributes associated with nursing are feminine characteristics.[1] While the percentage of men in the nursing profession has slowly increased over the past several decades, men in specialty areas such as labor and delivery, neonatal intensive care unit (NICU), midwifery, and pediatrics have not improved. In one study, the authors stated that in 2012, the percentage of male midwives was only 1%, which had remained constant for many years.[2] Many authors, in discussing men in highly female-dominated specialties, have urged for diversity within the workforce. These include child and adolescent mental health and midwifery.[3,4] Unfortunately, the numbers of men in these areas continue to be minimal.

[a] University of Alabama at Birmingham School of Nursing; [b] University of Wisconsin-Oshkosh College of Nursing, 800 Algoma Boulevard, Oshkosh, WI 54901, USA; [c] University of Wisconsin-Oshkosh College of Nursing
[1] Present address: W8385 Cloverleaf Lake Road, Clintonville, WI 54929, USA
* Corresponding author. NB446, 1720 2nd Avenue South, Birmingham, AL 35294.
*E-mail address:* cjborde@uab.edu

Nurs Clin N Am 58 (2023) 617–625
https://doi.org/10.1016/j.cnur.2023.06.005
nursing.theclinics.com

Oftentimes, male nursing students are not afforded experiences within these environments during nursing school. When they are, they tend to face isolation as well as feelings of anxiety, dread, or fear of rejection.[4] Male nursing students face sex-related bias in obstetric rotations as well as fear of suspect touch when caring for female clients.[4] Oftentimes, men will feel unwelcome in the clinical setting. There is a belief that the maternal-newborn clinical setting is inappropriate for male nursing students, while male physicians and medical students are perfectly acceptable.[5] Male students often experience nonsupportive clinical instructors and restrictions regarding care in the maternal-child rotation, causing them to feel they do not belong.[6,7] Gender bias has been reported, including male students placed in roles of observation, asked to leave the bedside without a patient requesting to do so, and denied the opportunity to observe deliveries on the maternal-newborn unit.[8] Authors of this article explore gender in nursing, a history of men in nursing, and concepts of men in female-dominated nursing specialty areas. A case study is provided of a male neonatal nurse practitioner working in the NICU.

## GENDER

Gender (in contrast to biological sex) refers to culturally defined roles and attributes associated with being or appearing to be a woman or a man; the gender binary refers to a system of considering and categorizing gender in which all people are either male or female.[9] While many people experience their gender identity as falling within these categories of "man" or "woman," others do not. In the 1990s, the term "genderqueer" emerged to describe someone who felt their gender lay outside of the binary, between male and female, or not completely identifying with one specific binary identity.[10] Genderqueer may be used as an umbrella term for any gender outside of "male" and "female" or may have a uniquely rebellious connotation as a challenge to the master gender binary narrative.[10] "Nonbinary" began to appear in the lexicon shortly after "genderqueer," and the broader and more inclusive term "gender diverse" is an even more recent term. Gender diverse has been defined as a term that recognizes that all people express and identify with a gender identity and that the identity and expression are not necessarily linked to a person's sexual characteristics.[10] Clinicians may be more familiar with the term "transgender," which describes people whose internal knowledge of their own gender does not align with the sex they were assigned at birth.[11,12] However, some nonbinary people do not identify as transgender and consequently may face discrimination from both outside and inside the transgender community.[13] While nonbinary people have always existed, research around nonbinary identities is extremely new and limited; as most research focuses on the transgender population, most clinicians have not been offered education on how to work with nonbinary people.[13]

## GENDER IN HEALTH CARE

The gender binary is a highly patriarchal system, assigning "greater value to men and things considered to be masculine than to women or things considered to be feminine" and "grant[ing] less legitimacy to gender identities or expressions that do not conform (p. 2441)".[9] Gender norms are the glue holding this system together. Gender norms can be defined as "social norms defining acceptable and appropriate actions for women and men in a given group or society. They are embedded in formal and informal institutions, nested in the mind, and produced and reproduced through social interaction (pp. 415–416)."[14] Restrictive gender norms and the pervasiveness of the gender binary have a significant impact on health outcomes, both for individuals who identify within the gender binary and those who do not.

Health systems reinforce gender norms, resulting in poorer outcomes for women, men, and gender minorities. Gender norms dictate men's and women's domains; for example, services for women are often focused on their reproductive and care-giving capacity, while at the same time, clinicians often resist men's engagement in maternal and pediatric care.[15] While women have higher risks than men for certain conditions, including depression, anxiety, cancer, and aging-related health burdens, they may receive worse care; stereotypes of women as fragile and emotional can lead to their health complaints being perceived as exaggerated or being attributed to psychosomatic causes.[9,16]

Gender norms around masculinity can lead to clinicians viewing men as strong, not needing care, and less compliant than female patients, despite men's lower life expectancy and many higher health risks relative to women.[16] Gender biases can be exacerbated when clinicians encounter patients who represent a gender or sexual minority. Nonbinary individuals face unique barriers in health care, many of which are not experienced by transgender people. Nonbinary people may experience worse mental health outcomes and higher rates of suicide than their binary transgender peers.[17] Gendered language and policies in health care settings, such as "reassigning" nonbinary patients within a binary gender, can create barriers, resulting in a breakdown of trust and unwillingness to seek needed care.[18,19] Consequently, nonbinary people and other gender minorities are more likely to delay care, putting them at risk of chronic health issues.[19] Nonbinary people may have difficulty accessing gender-affirming medical or surgical care if providers do not consider them to be truly transgender, as the dominant medical narrative requires a "transition" from one binary gender to another.[13,17]

## HISTORY OF MEN IN NURSING

When trying to define nursing from a historical perspective, a nurse can be viewed as a person who takes care of the sick, injured, and aged.[20] Based on this definition, a nurse is any individual who cares for others, usually occurring outside the home. Before the time of Nightingale, care of individuals outside of the home was viewed as unfit for women.[21] This means that men were usually the individuals providing nursing care to sick and injured individuals within the community.

As previously stated, men typically provided nursing care to outsiders. The first known people trained in nursing were men during the Hippocratic period of ancient Greece. These men served as assistants to the physician, while women often cared for those within the home. This was due to the role of society which banned women to the home.[22] The first recorded school of nursing was established in 250 B.C. in India.[23] In this school, only men were considered pure enough to become nurses. Men had served as nurses for many centuries until Nightingale created her schools of nursing.

The first time that a woman was mentioned as a nurse in the United States was in 1890.[23] In 1896, a delegate of 20 female nurses gather in New York City to form the Nurses Associated Alumnae of the United States and Canada.[24] This group, which became the American Nurses Association (ANA) in 1911, excluded men from joining its ranks.[1,24] It was not until 1930 that bylaws were amended to allow men to become members of the ANA (Nursingworld, nd). Men did not join the ANA until 1940.[25]

Men were excluded from attending nursing schools, except for the few nursing schools for men. In fact, in 1960, 85% of nursing schools excluded the admittance of men into their program based solely on their gender.[1]

In terms of military nursing, the Army Nurse Corp in the United States was formed in 1901 by and for women. It was the only branch of the military that women could serve in. These women were commissioned as nurses, while men, although receiving the same training, were relegated to the role of orderly.[25] Men were forbidden from being nurses in the Army Nurse Corp. With the allowance of men into the ANA in the 1930s and 1940s, there was increasing pressure for men to be allowed to practice in the ANC. In 1955, Congress passed legislation allowing men to join the U.S. Army Reserves for assignment into the ANC. Lieutenant Edward T. Lyon was the first male commissioned into the ANC.[26]

In 1966, Congress passed a law authorizing the commissioning of men into the ANC.[25] Also of note, in 2004, the Supreme Court ruled against a hospital policy that prevented men from working in the obstetrics unit.[1] This ruling is critical, as up until this point, men were often prevented from working in specialty areas. However, even with this ruling, men in nursing still face barriers in specialty areas. Many male nursing students faced differential treatment from both faculty and female patients when having clinicals in the maternity setting.

In a study conducted with midwives, in which men only constitute 1%, there are mixed opinions. Of the respondents, 71.4% believed that men belong in midwifery, while 74% felt that gender did not impact the quality of care.[2] While some participants viewed men's perspectives critical to midwifery's values of nondiscrimination, gender equality, and feminism, others felt that in order to provide care for a woman, the provider must be a woman. Many of the historical biases that have existed related to men in nursing were discussed by a small percentage of midwives.

These concerns related to a lack of trust of men in nursing. This minority questioned the motives of men who were midwives. They felt that men who wanted to be midwives were self-serving, less altruistic, or motivated by inappropriate sexual desires. What was demonstrated more was a conflict where midwives have values including inclusion and diversity but also wanted to keep midwifery a women-only space.[2] This example helps to demonstrate that men are still not viewed positively by all in many of the typically female-dominated specialty areas of nursing.

## DISCUSSION

Men continue to face bias in many areas of nursing practice. As was stated previously, the landscape of nursing changed with Nightengale's creation of her school of nursing. Before this time, nursing was viewed as a profession for the poor or classless in Europe. Nightingale wanted to change this perception by bringing middle- to upper-class white females into her schools and training them as nurses. One of the policies that she implemented in her schools of nursing was to not allow men into the program.[1] The only exception was for men to care where their strength was required. Even when they received training, this was subpar to what female students received. The area where their strength was required was in mental health institutions.[1] In fact, Nightingale was quoted as saying that "every woman is a nurse ... men have no place in nursing except where physical strength is needed" (KeithRN, 2019).

During this time period, Victorian separatist views of gender were at their strongest. Nightingale felt that nursing was natural for women and that by becoming a nurse, they were only doing what came naturally to them. In this viewpoint, along with her view of apprenticeship models of education, she believed that women did not require education before working in hospitals under the supervision of male physicians.

What this created was a family-based institutional model of health care. In this model, the physician was viewed as the father of the family. The nurse was viewed as the mother of the family. Finally, the patient was viewed as the child. In Victorian society, the mother was often subservient to the father. What this model created was that the nurse was subservient to the physician. It also created a sense that men did not belong in nursing as it would upset the family dynamic of father, mother, and children.

This viewpoint has continued in the nursing profession. Oftentimes, men are excluded from working in areas or are called up to help lift a patient. While nurses continue to fight for equality and autonomy, many of the perceptions of nurse as handmaiden to the physician continue. Without having this model during the creation of the modern nursing profession, nursing could be in a completely different place in terms of power and having a voice from where it is today.

## Men in Nursing Specialties

In recent years, more and more men are entering the nursing profession. According to the American Association of Colleges of Nursing, approximately 14% of entry-level nurses identify as male.[27] Male nurses are capable of performing the same duties as their female counterparts such as providing patient care, administering medication, monitoring vital signs, and communicating with care providers of the interprofessional team. Men choose to enter the nursing profession for a variety of reasons. A systematic review revealed four main themes of why men pursued nursing: early exposure to nursing, by chance, extrinsic factors (job security, salary, opportunities), and intrinsic factors (personal satisfaction and enjoyment).[28] These factors influence male perception of nursing and the growing acceptance of men in the field.

Male nurses can work in a variety of health care settings such as hospitals, clinics, long-term care facilities, and home health agencies. Male nurses traditionally fill roles within adult intensive and acute care environments; however, opportunities exist in all settings. It is important to note that male nurses face some unique challenges in their profession. Male nurses may face challenges of discrimination or bias from colleagues or patients based on their gender.[29,30] Patients may feel uncomfortable with a male caring for them based on gender. According to Kronsberg and colleagues,[29] male nurses experience discrimination among colleagues, a lack of support from family and friends, and dissatisfaction in the educational and clinical practice environments. Male nurses were seen as uncaring, unable to empathize with family needs, and unapproachable. By discussing the value of men in nursing, we can aid in reducing bias and normalize a diverse workforce.

Male nurses can make a significant contribution to nursing and the health care field. Male nurses are an important and valuable part of any health care team, including those working in the NICU. Evidence is lacking on male nurses in the NICU. The presence of male nurses in the NICU is increasingly recognized as a positive aspect of patient care by providing a unique and diverse perspective and skillset to the interprofessional care team.[30] Male nurses can provide unique emotional support to families and colleagues in the often high-stress setting of the NICU. Parents may feel more comfortable discussing their experience with male nurses about certain issues or concerns. Male nurses can provide a different type of empathy and support, beneficial for families going through the emotional experience of having a baby in the NICU. Fathers of babies in the NICU often feel disconnected and unable to "care" for the family.[31,32] By increasing the male presence within the NICU, fathers may feel more connected and involved in the baby's care. Ultimately, having a diverse and inclusive team of health care providers, including male nurses, is important for ensuring the best possible care for patients and their families.

## A Case Study of an NICU Experience

An author within this work has first-hand knowledge and experience of being a male nurse in the neonatal ICU.

I am from a family- and faith-centric, small town in central Louisiana. At the time, I was a first-generation college student. I always felt connected with helping others. From volunteering to help family and friends with projects to restoring my first car, I had a passion to collaborate and grow. I never thought my path would take me to caring for infants, but I can reflect on an amazing and fulfilling career. My first experience within the neonatal ICU was as a final semester student in a bachelorette nursing program. During our final semester, students select an area of interest for a final practicum experience. I selected the neonatal ICU. At first, many of my student colleagues asked, "why do you want to work in the NICU"? But once I began learning more about caring for the smallest and most vulnerable patients, I was convinced I was in the right environment. From medications, to procedures, to the often-complex family situations, I found the NICU environment to be both challenging and rewarding. I absorbed as much knowledge as I could and asked for the most critical infants. I felt connected to the patients and families and truly felt I was making a difference. I was professional and personally fulfilled and believed the perfect path was taken. However, it was not always roses.

Discrimination, unwelcoming comments, lack of trust from families, and profiling were experienced during my career. More-experienced female nurses would ask, "why do you want to be in here," "men have no place in the NICU ... this is for moms and grandmothers," "you don't know the first thing about caring for people ... you are a man." I would often receive undesirable assignments, would not be asked to lunch, and watched as I interacted with breastfeeding mothers. All this took a toll on me, and I started to second guess my place in the NICU. And then I had a male neonatal nurse practitioner tell me, "ignore them ... they did that to me too. They don't think we should be here." He gave the best advice ever ... learn as much as you can and prove that you know what you are doing." I accepted the challenge and never looked back. I became certified as a neonatal nurse, completed a graduate degree as a neonatal nurse practitioner, and ultimately completed a doctoral degree. As a nurse practitioner, I learned every skill I could and made time to teach others. Nurses want to feel they are learning and the best way to care for their babies. I feel connected to the family as a whole, with fathers and male parents asking me more questions and wanting to be more included. By making the time to share my knowledge and experience, I empowered more nurses to do the same. It is hard to overcome bias, profiling, and discrimination. Our power to do so comes from within.

## CLINICAL IMPLICATIONS

With the increasing presence of men in nursing, the profession is becoming more diverse, resulting in challenges to traditional gender roles and stereotypes. This diversification promotes a more inclusive, creative, and patient-focused health care environment. By diversifying the nursing workforce, there is a potential to enhance patient comfort and satisfaction. Patients may find it easier to communicate with male counterparts, resulting in more comprehensive patient care. The presence of men in the nursing workforce expands the scope of health care services such as men's health clinics and men's primary care services. If male nurses and advanced-level nurses are available in primary care clinics, then male patients may be more willing to seek preventative services. The increased availability of diverse to-care services can help address disparities in health care and improve overall health outcomes for men. Men in nursing can serve as role models and mentors for nursing students and experienced nurses. The presence of male nurses challenges the prevailing notion that nursing is exclusively a female-dominated environment. By sharing their experiences, as within this article, male nurses can inspire others and contribute to the recruitment and retention of more men in nursing.

## SUMMARY

Men often are the subject of bias and marginalization within the nursing profession. This has occurred since the creation of the modern nursing profession by Florence Nightingale. While men have made inroads into the profession, having seen increased numbers in many areas, men still face many challenges in working in many specialty areas. These areas typically involve the care of women and children, such as labor and delivery, NICU, and pediatric units.

However, men bring a unique perspective to the environment. They can better relate to things that husbands, boyfriends, and fathers are going through. They can explain things in a way that the men will understand. They also provide empathetic, high-quality care to all their patients, just like their female counterparts do. It is important to understand the different means of caregiving that men bring to the profession. It is also critical to understand that neither way of providing care is good or bad. They are just different. In understanding and embracing the differences that all individuals bring to the profession, nursing can deliver the individualized, person-centered care that has been talked about for generations but can never be fully realized without having a diverse workforce.

## CLINICS CARE POINTS

- Diversification of the nurisng workforce promotes a more inclusive, creative, and patient-focused health care environment.
- Men in nursing can serve as role models and mentors for nursing students and experienced nurses.

## DISCLOSURES

The authors have nothing to disclose.

## REFERENCES

1. KeithRN. Men in nursing. 2019. Available at: https://www.keithrn.com/2019/02/men-in-nursing/. Accessed May 22, 2023.
2. Bly K, Ellis SA, Ritter RJ, et al. A survey of midwives' attitudes toward men in midwifery. J Midwifery Womens Health 2020;65(2):199–207.
3. Holyoake D-D. Similarly different: exploring how male nurses in CAMHS experience difference in their gender performance. Compr Child Adolesc Nurs 2020; 43(4):389–409.
4. MacWilliams B, Schmidt B, Bleich M. Men in nursing. AJN The American Journal of Nursing 2013;113(1):38–44.
5. Akpuaka S, Clarke-Tasker V. A qualitative study to explore the male nursing student's coping with experiences in a maternal-newborn nursing course. J Natl Black Nurses Assoc 2017;28. 31-17.
6. Eswi A, El-Sayed Y. The experience of Egyptian male student nurses during attending maternity nursing clinical course. Nur Educ Practice 2011;11(2):93–8.

7. Sedgwick M, Kellett P. Exploring masculinity and marginalization of male undergraduate nursing students' experience of belonging during clinical experiences. J Nurs Educ 2015;54(3):121–9.

8. Carnevale T, Priode K. "The good ole' girls' nursing club": the male student perspective. J Transcult Nurs 2018;29:285–91.

9. Heise N, Greene ME, Opper N, et al. Gender inequality and restrictive gender norms: framing the challenges to health. Lancet 2019;393(10189):2440–54.

10. Thorne N, Yip AK, Bouman WP, et al. The terminology of identities between, outside and beyond the gender binary - A systematic review. Int J Transgenderism 2019;20(2–3):138–54.

11. GLAAD. GLAAD Transgender Media Program. 2023. Available at: https://www.glaad.org/transgender. Accessed May 22, 2023.

12. Streed CG Jr, Navarra M, Klein J. Advancing undergraduate medical education regarding the care of transgender and gender Diverse persons and communities. Perspect Med Educ 2022;11(6):306–8.

13. National LGBT Health Education Center. Providing Affirmative Care for Patients with Non-binary Gender Identities. 2016. Available at: https://www.lgbtqiahealtheducation.org/wp-content/uploads/2017/02/Providing-Affirmative-Care-for-People-with-Non-Binary-Gender-Identities.pdf. Accessed May 22, 2023.

14. Cislaghi B, Heise L. Gender norms and social norms: differences, similarities and why they matter in prevention science. Sociol Health Illn 2020;42(2):407–22.

15. Gupta GR, Oomman N, Grown C, et al. Gender equality and gender norms: framing the opportunities for health. Lancet 2019;393(10190):2550–62.

16. Smith DT, Mouzon DM, Elliott M. Reviewing the assumptions about men's mental health: an exploration of the gender binary. Am J Men's Health 2018;12(1):78–89.

17. Matsuno E, Budge SL. Non-binary/Genderqueer Identities: a critical review of the literature. Curr Sex Health Rep 2017;9(3):116–20.

18. Durocher K, Caxaj CS. Gender binaries in nursing: a critical shift to postgenderism. Nurs Womens Health 2022;26(4):262–8.

19. Hsieh N, Shuster SM. Health and health care of sexual and gender minorities. J Health Soc Behav 2021;62(3):318–33.

20. Ellis JR, Hartley CL. Nursing in today's world: trends, issues & management. Philadelphia: Lippincott Williams & Wilkins; 2004.

21. D'Antonio P, Buhler-Wilkerson K. Nursing. 2019. Available at: https://www.britannica.com/science/nursing#ref36766. Accessed May 22, 2023.

22. O'Lynn CE, Tranbarger RE. Men in nursing: history, challenges, and opportunities. New York, NY: Springer; 2007.

23. Howard G. What do you know about the history of nursing? The Alabama Nurse. 2008. Available at: https://www.abn.alabama.gov/wp-content/uploads/2016/02/2008-abn-annual-report.pdf. Accessed May 22, 2023.

24. American Nurses Association. The history of the American nurses association. n.d. Available at: https://www.nursingworld.org/ana/about-ana/history/. Accessed May 22, 2023.

25. Carleton E. Nurse Corps fought to include male nurses as officers. 2019. Available at: https://www.army.mil/article/216814/nurse_corps_fought_to_include_male_nurses_as_officers. Accessed May 22, 2023.

26. Lotts L. Men in nursing: History, stereotypes, and the gender pay gap. 2019. Available at: https://www.onlinefnpprograms.com/features/men-in-nursing/. Accessed May 22, 2023.

27. American Association of Colleges of Nursing. Fact Sheet: Enhancing Diversity in the Nursing Workforce. 2020. Available at: https://www.aacnnursing.org/Portals/42/News/Factsheets/Enhancing-Diversity-Factsheet.pdf. Accessed May 22, 2023.

28. Yi M, Keogh B. What motivates men to choose nursing as a profession? A systematic review of qualitative studies. Contemp Nurse 2014;52(1):95–105.

29. Kronsberg S, Bouret R, Brett A. Lived experiences of male nurses: dire consequences for the nursing profession. J Nur Educ Practice 2018;8(1):46–53.

30. Mohammadi F, Oshvandi K, Med HK. Male nursing students' perception of dignity in neonatal intensive care units. Nurs Ethics 2020;27(2):381–9.

31. Feeley N, Sherrard K, Waitzer E, et al. The father at the bedside. J Perinat Neonatal Nurs 2013;27(1):72–80.

32. Hearn C, Clarkson G, Day M. The role of the NICU in father involvement, beliefs, and confidence. Nat Assoc Neo Nur 2019;20(1):80–9.

# Consideration of Gender on Hormone Therapy Management

Lindsay L. Morgan, DNP, FNP-BC

## KEYWORDS

- Hormone therapy • Risk factors • Male • Female • Transgender • Gender diverse
- Gender-inclusive • Hormone therapy similarities

## KEY POINTS

- Common risks in both women and transgender and gender-diverse women with the use of hormone therapy.
- Common risks in both men and transgender and gender-diverse men with the use of hormone therapy.
- Commonalities in screening and management among cisgender and transgender individuals are notable.
- Gender-inclusive screening for risks is needed in clinical practice guidelines for hormone therapy initiation and management.
- Lack of inclusion of transgender and gender-diverse individuals in hormone therapy studies causes a clinical gap for provider guidance in hormone therapy risks and monitoring for this population.

## INTRODUCTION

Hormone replacement therapy (HRT) or hormone therapy (HT) has been known since antiquity. Estrogen therapy has been available since the 1960s used primarily to treat menopause with clinical trials of HRT beginning in the 1990s.[1] Testosterone therapy began in the 1930s and was initially used to treat primary hypogonadism.[2] Since the documented use of sex hormone therapy, science has expanded, advanced, and refined the use of sex hormone therapy to offer comprehensive coverage for additional medical needs in males, females, and transgender and gender-diverse (TGD) individuals. In this document, the HT discussion will consist of its use in the management of menopausal symptoms, secondary hypogonadism, or late-onset hypogonadism in adults, and gender-affirming care in TGD adults. The hormone therapy treatment

The author declares no conflict of interest.
University of Wisconsin Oshkosh, College of Nursing, 800 Algoma Boulevard, Oshkosh, WI 54901, USA
*E-mail address:* morganl@uwosh.edu

0029-6465/23/© 2023 Elsevier Inc. All rights reserved.

methods among these groups have notable similarities and differences. A gender-inclusive approach to research involves participants of different gender identities analyzed as one heterogenous population rather than different gender identities analyzed as separate groups.[3] Gender-inclusivity in HT management needs recognition in research and clinical practice guidelines to improve hormone therapy management strategies in clinical practice to optimize patient outcomes.

Developing awareness of gender-inclusive hormone therapy management means providers must also develop understanding of the distinct differences between sex and gender and the expression of gender transition. Gender and sex are two distinctly different terms. Sex refers to biological attributes associated with physical and physiologic features including chromosomes, gene expression, hormone function and level, and reproductive anatomy of men, women, and TGD individuals while gender traditionally refers to socially constructed characteristics such as norms, roles, and relations.[4] There is conflicting evidence, however, listing gender identity as including an innate biologic component in humans, rather than a reversible trait developed from societal constructs.[5] There are additional terms that providers need to be cognizant of when providing HT treatment and management. A cisgender person's gender identity and assigned sex at birth match.[6] Transgender and gender diverse are terms used to describe a person whose gender identity and assigned sex at birth do not match.[7] Gender transition involves the adoption of characteristics that match the individual's gender identity. This can mean changing hair, clothing, and identity documents or changing physical appearance with HT and/or surgical intervention.[6] TGD men and women may use the term "man" or woman" when referring to themselves. For the purpose of differentiation in this document, TGD will be used when referring to individuals whose gender identity is different from their assigned sex at birth.

Genetics, regardless of sex and gender at the time of HT initiation, is another provider consideration in HT management. There is genetic variation in every individual that contributes to disease risk, making most diseases heritable. Genetic heritability is the likelihood of genetic expression. The likelihood of the presentation of personal characteristics or chronic diseases occurs as a result of genetic heritability. The genetic heritability of height and pubertal timing is between 50% and 80%. Serum lipid levels have a 40% to 60% change of being influenced by genetics. The probability of developing common chronic disease based on genetics is as follows: type 1 diabetes mellitus (DM) is up to 80%, type 2 DM is between 40% and 80%, obesity is 40% to 70%, hypertension (HTN) 30% to 70%, and osteoporosis 50% to 85%.[8] It is also known that the onset of menopause, development of breast cancer, development of cardiovascular disease (CVD), and presence of thrombophilias have a genetic component. Genetic heritability, regardless of sex or gender, explains the need to consider genetic predisposition to diseases prior to the initiation of hormone therapy. Providers must assess all facets of a patient's health profile including sex at birth, gender, personal social and medical history, and family history in order to determine if HT is appropriate for the patient.

Genetics also plays a role in sex and sex development. At the very early stages of fetal development there are biological sex-related changes that occur. Historically, it was thought there were two sexes with XY and XX chromosomes, however there are many different variations of sex-specific chromosomes and the genes that differentiate and determine sex. As a result, patients can present with underlying conditions that vary in severity, have ambiguous genitalia, or have no obvious alteration in genitalia at birth, but have the external genitalia be incongruent with internal sex processes.[9] Data suggest a biologic underpinning with associations between brain anatomy and gender identity.[10] These considerations imply patients with TGD may have variable sex-specific cells, independent of secondary sex characteristics visible at birth and HT may influence the patient based on their sex-specific cells.[9] More research is needed in this area.

As a result of individual chromosomal makeup, genetics, and sex-specific cells, the body secretes hormones. Transportation of hormones is a unique homeostatic state for all people. Gonadal hormone synthesis is achieved by the homeostatic function of the hypothalamic-pituitary-gonadal axis. Hypothalamic and pituitary cells monitor circulating hormone concentrations and secrete trophic hormones, which activate specific pathways for hormone synthesis and release.[11] HT may be a consideration for all sexes and genders, based on individual needs, because all people have receptors that will respond to testosterone and estrogen.[12]

In females, there is coordinated function between the hypothalamus, pituitary gland, ovaries and endometrium to allow the physiologic process of ovulation and menstruation. The hypothalamus secretes gonadotropin-releasing hormone (GnRH) stimulating the anterior pituitary gland to secrete follicle-stimulating hormone (FSH) and luteinizing hormone (LH). Sex hormones, estrogen (estradiol), progesterone, and ovarian peptides along with pituitary follistatin modify the secretion of FSH and LH, allowing for hormone fluctuation to influence the sex-specific organs and to manage the cycle of ovulation and menstruation.[13] It is known that estrogen not only acts on the reproductive organs, but also on the cardiovascular organs, and bone, among others.[14]

Like females, the control of testosterone in males is through the secretion of GnRH from the hypothalamus which stimulates the pituitary gland to secrete FSH and LH. LH acts on the Leydig cells of the testes to stimulate testosterone production. With the help of FSH, testosterone then works locally in the testicles to promote spermatogenesis. Testosterone is also secreted into the circulation where it works on many other body tissues. This complete process is known as the hypothalamic–pituitary–testicular axis.[15]

Considering what is known about sex, gender identity, genetics, and hormone transport, it is appropriate to state that an individual treatment plan with a gender-inclusive approach is needed for patients who are interested in HT for medical needs such as menopause or hypogonadism or for gender-affirming needs. Understanding the current determination for HT along with treatment and monitoring methodology for the above problems will undrape the commonalities and determine the level of gender inclusivity that is feasible.

## Discussion

### Clinical relevance

**Hormone therapy use in cisgender women.** Hormone therapy for the management of menopausal symptoms in cisgender women has been widely used for many years. The use of HT has markedly decreased since a 2002 study was released by the Writing Group for Women's Health Initiative Investigators (WHI) concluding the risks of HT outweigh the benefits. This study instilled fears of breast cancer and heart attacks that were found to be misinterpreted by the data for over 2 decades. On the contrary, additional research found if HT is initiated before the age of 60 or within 10 years of menopause, it is thought to be health-protective in some ways, reducing mortality and risk of coronary disease, osteoporosis, and dementias while lack of HT can cause increased risk of chronic diseases and mortality.[16] The International Menopause Society's 2016 recommendations conclude that the most recent Cochrane analysis, other meta-analyses, and the follow up, 13-year results of WHI show a consistent reduction in all-cause mortality in women starting HT (with or without progestogen) under

60 years of age and/or within 10 years of menopause.[17] However, there remains conflicting evidence for the individual risk of cardiovascular disease, stroke, venous thromboembolism (VTE), and breast cancer development with the consideration of existing risk factors and the type, timing, dosing, duration, and formulation of estrogen and/or progestogen therapy used. HT is currently not recommended as a means of disease prevention therapy.[18] Nonetheless, it has been determined by several prominent medical societies since the 2002 WHI study, that estrogen therapy is appropriate for younger, healthy women at the onset of or within 10 years of menopause and in most cases, the benefits outweigh the risks. The use of estrogen in postmenopausal women is being explored as an emerging possibility.[19]

Recognizing the cardiovascular and neurovascular risks and benefits associated with estrogen therapy, with or without progestogen, and with the consideration of the route of estrogen, is essential for comprehensive menopausal management. Menopausal HT has several benefits related to CVD. A reduction in atherosclerosis progression, coronary heart disease, and cardiovascular-related deaths was observed with the use of HT when initiated before age 60 or within 10 years of menopause. Additionally, current evidence reveals there is no increase in cardiovascular events or mortality in women when HT was initiated 10 or more years after menopause.[18,20] VTE and stroke development are potential risks with the use of HT is dependent upon the route of administration (oral vs transdermal) and other predisposing risk factors such as obesity, immobility, age, personal or family history of VTE, hereditary thrombophilia's, and immobility. Oral estrogen therapy has been shown to increase the risk of strokev.[18] Based on these factors, the initiation and management of HT are dependent upon an individualized assessment by the clinician.

Providers must evaluate patients for a personal or family history of cancer when considering the use of HT in a treatment plan due to HT's potential cancer-causing effects. It has been found that breast, endometrial, and ovarian cancer risk is increased in HT users while a reduction in cervical, liver, and colorectal cancer has been observed.[21] There are many factors that influence cancer risk and cancer reduction in correlation to the use of HT including types and formulations of estrogen and progestogen, dosing, duration, timing of initiation, combination therapy, and personal risk factors such as body mass index (BMI) and physical activity level, current CVD, tobacco and alcohol use, other lifestyle factors, and family history of cancer.[21] However, current evidence concludes estrogen-only HT, has little to no increased risk of breast cancer, specifically, in patients without known breast cancer. Patients with known breast cancer should avoid oral estrogen. Combined HT appears to pose an increased risk of breast cancer dependent upon the duration of therapy.[18] More research is needed regarding HT use and the development of breast and other cancers.

Menopause is also plagued by many changes including vasomotor symptoms, depression, anxiety, and cognitive decline, which can have an immense alteration on quality of life. Hot flashes and night sweats are two common vasomotor symptoms that occur during menopause that can affect sleep, causing mood changes and anxiety. Depression can occur in menopausal women due to an interaction between the estrogen and serotonin transmitter pathway. Sexual desire, libido, and cognition can diminish during menopause. HT has been reported to improve these symptoms in menopausal patients.[18]

Metabolic changes and deterioration of bone tissue are other common occurrences due to menopause. Lack of estrogen contributes to insulin resistance and decreased glucose tolerance increasing the risk for DM development in menopausal women. HT improves insulin resistance, increases glucose tolerance, and reduces the new onset of DM by 20%–30% (20 Hodis). The risk of osteoporosis in menopausal women is attributed to the lack of estrogen, causing altered bone remodeling and intervertebral disc thinning. The use of HT has been shown to reduce bone turnover and increase bone mass thus decreasing the risk of osteoporosis or further decrease in bone mineral density (BMD).[22]

Providers must first assess if HT is appropriate for the menopausal patient by completing a thorough history and physical. Determining age, obesity, mood, presence of vasomotor symptoms, potential for high –risk endometrial cancer or a history of breast cancer, CVD, VTE, stroke, or transient ischemic attack will influence the decision to initiate HT and steer the treatment plan. Additionally, determining the presence of influential lifestyle factors and cardiovascular risk calculation less than 10% 10-year risk using a CVD risk calculator tool can be part of the initial evaluation.[19,23] After discussing the risks and benefits with the patient, an informed decision can be made. Treatment varies and is dependent upon patient history and menopausal symptoms. Treatment monitoring and screening vary depending on other morbidities and medications. The United States Preventative Services Task Force (USPSTF) recommends screening for prediabetes and DM in adults aged 35 to 70 who are overweight or have obesity.[24] USPSTF recommends biennial mammography for women 50 to 74. Screening for 40 to 49 year old women is recommended if they have a parent, child, or sibling with breast cancer.[25] Mammography is not recommended more frequently for individuals using HT with no additional breast cancer risk. Increased breast cancer monitoring would be dependent on the individual.[23]

Lastly, it is with consensus from most studies and supporting organizations, that the initiation, monitoring, and continuation of HT in menopausal cisgender women requires an individualized approach with the consideration of individual risks and benefits.[19] It is also with consensus that once deemed appropriate, menopausal HT is considered safe and effective with a greater benefit versus risk in improving quality of life if administered before age 60 or within 10 years of menopause.[18] Additionally, it is thought there is no need to place arbitrary, mandatory treatment duration limits on HT if patients participate in ongoing reassessment and reevaluation of risks and benefits of therapy, however research on long-term effects and safety of estrogen therapy is lacking.[16]

**Hormone therapy use in cisgender men.** Hormone therapy for the management of hypogonadism has been widely used for many years. Testosterone is the primary hormone used to treat a range of signs related to secondary, functional testosterone deficiency, or late-onset hypogonadism (LOH), such as decreased libido, erectile dysfunction, depressed mood, anemia, and loss of muscle and bone mass.[26] The primary causes of LOH include obesity, type 2 diabetes, or metabolic syndrome. Along with lifestyle changes, men can benefit from testosterone therapy in many ways including improved sexual function, improved mood and sense of well-being, increased BMD, and increased muscle mass, strength, and function.[27] Cardioprotective benefits of testosterone therapy have not been thoroughly studied with one study showing a decrease in total cholesterol and low-density lipoprotein, while other studies showed increased risk of cardiac-related events such as myocardial infarction and stroke.[28] Like menopausal females, bone density changes occur in males over time and osteoporosis may develop due to the associated androgen changes and testosterone declines. There are other contributing conditions and lifestyle factors that contribute to osteoporosis development including smoking or alcohol use, glucocorticoid excess, and idiopathic hypercalcemia.[22] BMD has been shown to improve in the lumbar spine after approximately 6 months of testosterone therapy, showing a benefit of its use.[27]

There are several risks associated with testosterone use that must be considered prior to HT initiation. Testosterone therapy causes increased circulating red blood cells (RBC), known as erythrocytosis, due to testosterone's stimulating effects on RBC production in the bone marrow. Erythrocytosis can increase blood viscosity and cause or worsen CVD and VTE development. Testosterone can also cause fluid retention and edema, which can potentially exacerbate congestive heart failure (CHF) or other edematous conditions.[27] Because of this, testosterone is contraindicated in men with thrombophilia, unstable CVD, uncontrolled heart failure, severe, untreated heart failure or ischemia, stroke, or recent (within 3–6 months) cardiovascular events. Erythrocytosis and the resultant increased risk of thrombosis, occurs more often in older men.[27] Mild to severe lower urinary tract symptoms (LUTS) caused by benign prostatic hyperplasia (BPH) may be considered a contraindication for testosterone use. History of obstructive sleep apnea (OSA) or severe, untreated OSA, and men who desire fertility in the next 6 to 12 months are additional contraindications to HT.[26] Testosterone therapy is contraindicated in men with breast cancer, locally advanced or metastatic prostate cancer, or those with palpable prostate nodules without treatment due to high risk of serious adverse outcomes.[27]

Monitoring for therapeutic response and screening for associated risks of testosterone HT should occur incrementally. A baseline serum testosterone and hematocrit level would be checked as part of the initial workup for late-onset hypogonadism. Additional testosterone levels would be completed at 3 months and again at 6 months during the first year of therapy. Levels would then be monitored every 6 to 12 months, thereafter. Hematocrit would be measured at 3 months, 6 months, 12 months, and annually.[26] Assessing for HT side effects and goals of therapy will be completed at approximately 3 months, 12 months, and then annually and as needed. Screening for prostate cancer by measuring the prostate-specific antigen (PSA) would occur after 3 months and again after 6 months of therapy for men 55 to 69 years of age with a prostate. For men younger than 55 with an increased risk of prostate cancer, screening would occur at the same increments. For men older than 69 years of age it is recommended to follow current prostate cancer screening guidelines. After 1 year of testosterone therapy, current prostate cancer screening guidelines would also be followed. BMD should be monitored after 1 to 2 years of therapy only if it was determined that a baseline BMD was needed and was found to be low.[26]

Recommendations for long-term HT use in men are based on limited randomized control trials, non-randomized clinical studies, and observational studies and do not include long-term effects on chronic conditions or new onset of conditions. It is recommended that clinicians promote individualized care while considering the patient's unique health history and morbidities in the initiation and management of male HT to optimize outcomes and improve quality of life.[26]

**Hormone therapy use in transgender and gender-diverse women.** TGD women may elect to complete transfeminine HT as part of gender transition. Transfeminine hormone therapy goals include reduction in body and facial hair growth, induction of breast development, and induction of female-patterned fat and muscle redistribution.[10] HT for TGD women generally includes estrogen (in the form of estradiol), testosterone-inhibiting drugs and progesterone as the commonly used gender affirming hormone therapy (GAHT) treatment options. However, the use of progesterone as part of the treatment plan in patients using GAHT requires further research to determine effects and recommendations for length of use.[29] The risks and benefits of transfeminine HT are comparable to the risks and benefits of menopausal HT. The route of estrogen is relevant to the risk of VTE development over time based on personal, existing, or history of thrombophilic conditions or family history of heritable thrombophilic conditions.[29] Contraindications to HT for TGD women include the history of breast cancer, history of or current VTE, CVD or cerebrovascular disease. As a result of the known coagulating effects of estrogen, and the potential hypercoagulable factors of the individual, all patients should be informed of the risk as well as screened for personal or family VTE history, smoking, or active malignancy before the initiation of transfeminine HT. Although there is an association with VTE development and estrogen therapy, there is not a higher risk of myocardial infarction or transient ischemic attack among TGD individuals compared to cisgender individuals.[5] Data of estrogen therapy use in TGD women are lacking and there is no evidence related to mood changes, depression, or well-being for TGD individuals treated with HT.

HT for TGD women typically requires combination therapy of estrogen and/or progesterone and androgen-lowering drugs to achieve desired affects. Spironolactone and GnRH agonists such as leuprolide or goserelin acetate, and progestins such as cyproterone can be used as adjunct androgen-lowering therapy. Estrogen for transgender women is widely available in oral formulation of conjugated estrogen and 17-beta estradiol. Estrogen is available orally, topically, or intramuscularly. The route of estrogen is relevant to the risk of VTE development along with the duration of use as well as personal or family history of thrombophilic conditions.[29] If spironolactone is used as adjunct therapy, potassium levels should be monitored, because spironolactone is a potassium-sparing diuretic. Side effects of spironolactone include urinary frequency, hyperkalemia, and orthostatic hypotension. Feminizing physical changes, lowered serum testosterone levels, and prevention of elevated serum estrogen levels are the goals of combination HT for TGD individuals. Physical changes typically begin within the first several months and include decreased libido with spontaneous erections, decreased facial and body hair growth, muscle atrophy, redistribution of body fat to waist and hips, and gynecomastia.[5]

Monitoring of serum testosterone and estrogen levels occurs approximately every 3 months during the first year of treatment and every 6 to 12 months for the remainder of treatment with the goal of falling testosterone levels to less than 100 ng/dL and estrogen levels under 200 ng/dL. Routine screening for cancer based on present organs (eg, testicles, prostate, breast), osteoporosis, and CVD should be completed on an individual basis based on the patient's unique characteristics and screening guidelines.[5]

**Hormone therapy use in transgender and gender-diverse men.** TGD men may elect to complete transmasculine hormone therapy. The goals of transmasculine therapy generally include menstruation cessation, deepening of the voice, increase in body and facial hair growth, increased muscle mass, and redistribution of fat away from the waist and hips.[10] Transmasculine therapy primarily consists of testosterone as the GAHT. The associated risks of GAHT for GD men are like those of cisgender men using testosterone for LOH. Research on mood changes, depression, or well-being for TGD men treated with HT is lacking.

The risks for TGD men and HT use include erythrocytosis that can be exacerbated by preexisting conditions such as OSA, unknown thrombophilia, or lifestyle factors such as smoking. An observational study in older, cisgender men using testosterone therapy suggests patients with unrecognized thrombophilias are at an increased risk of VTE development.[29] However, a large cohort study and a meta-analysis of VTE risk in transgender men using GAHT demonstrated no concern for increased risk, compared to cisgender men using testosterone HT.[30]

Testosterone would be contraindicated in people who are pregnant, present with symptoms of unstable coronary artery disease, or those who have untreated erythrocytosis. Although there is no known increased risk of uterine or ovarian cancer with testosterone therapy, routine screening for cancer based on present organs (eg, cervical, breast) should be followed based on current cancer screening guidelines. There is conflicting literature regarding the risk of breast cancer and testosterone therapy in TGD men. Limited studies and case reports are available for men and TGD men regarding breast cancer development while on testosterone treatment. Of the limited studies, 4 cases were cisgender men, and 18 cases were transgender men ranging from 18 to 61 years of age. Testosterone treatment duration ranged weeks up to 25 years. There is limited data within the studies to determine if the breast cancer development and stage is related to testosterone and/or is dose dependent. Additional research is needed for the use of HT in TGD men. Currently, only informed decision-making is required as guidance for the initiation of testosterone HT in TGD men.[31] BMD and CVD screening should be completed on an individual basis based on the patient's unique characteristics and current screening guidelines.[5]

Testosterone levels would be expected to be in the range of 300 to 1000 ng/dL for cisgender men and TGD men receiving HT, regardless of the cause of low testosterone. Routine serum testosterone, hemoglobin, and hematocrit monitoring should be approximately every 3 months for the first year and every 6 to 12 months for the duration of therapy. Assessing for HT side effects and goals of treatment will also be completed at 3 months, 12 months, and then annually. Signs of male sexual maturation begin within several months after initiating testosterone therapy. Testosterone can be administered transdermally, subcutaneously, and orally. TGD men often use lower doses of testosterone than cisgender men due to smaller body mass.[5] Lastly, data is inadequate to determine an age when GAHT is considered unsafe or unnecessary.[30]

## SUMMARY

HT is an ever-evolving branch of medicine affecting all genders and consideration of gender-specific and gender-inclusive risk factors, along with management strategies is necessary for a holistic care approach. Understanding gender-inclusive risk factor stratification and providing gender-inclusive treatment can improve patient outcomes and reduce gender disparities. Providers need to focus on an individualized approach to HT to improve quality of life, while prioritizing safety and risk prevention and tailoring routine and intermittent screening and treatment plans to the individual. Gender-inclusive medicine will increase access for the minority gender groups and improve outcomes.

It is important that TGD individuals have equal access to medical research benefits and are not denied or explicitly excluded from clinical trials. Limited studies exist to define risks and benefits of long-term GAHT. The scarcity of evidence-based treatment guidelines, long-term safety studies on GAHT, and guidance for complex patient cases cause barriers in care.[12] The use of gender-inclusive studies and clinical trials will ensure results are generalizable for all sexes which can lead to effective, patent-centered treatment plans and improved patient outcomes. Additionally, gender-specific medicine and research, overall, are lacking in specialized research in the topics of women's health, men's health, and the health of TGD individuals. Pharmaceutical companies do have specialized biotech in the reproductive health of women and to a much smaller extent, men and TGD individuals. The available biotech is based primarily on the endocrine system without considering more specifically sex, gender, and genetics in the pharmacokinetics, pharmacodynamics, and bioavailability of hormone therapy to offer a more gender-inclusive approach to medicine and treatment modalities.[32]

Further research is needed to identify and understand sex and gender differences related to hormone therapy to develop a gender-inclusive approach to risk assessment, screening, and management strategies. Clinical trial results are used to guide practice, and it is important that these results can be applied to gender-diverse patient populations. Long-term effects of GAHT as well as HT use in cisgender men and women is not well known. More research is needed on the effects and outcomes of long-term HT use in all genders to improve gender-inclusive care.

## CLINICS CARE POINTS

- Common Screening and Risks Related to Estrogen Therapy between Women and TGD Women: Providers need to consider the commonalities of actual or potential risks and potential for underlying conditions before the initiation of estrogen therapy among cisgender and transgender women. Baseline screening includes age, obesity, immobility and personal or family history of CVD, stroke, VTE, thrombophilia, smoking or alcohol use, and breast or reproductive organ cancer. Screening for osteoporosis or metabolic disorder would also need to be considered based on personal or family history prior to HT commencement.[20,22] Following additional current screening recommendations based on individual and diverse backgrounds related to age, presence of reproductive organs, family and personal history, and lifestyle factors will assist clinical decision-making in the use and management of HT to avoid potential adverse effects.

- Management and Monitoring of Estrogen Therapy in Women and TGD Women: A common HT management theme in cisgender and transgender women is avoidance of oral estrogen, if possible, in those women with a high baseline VTE risk.[18] Monitoring serum hormone levels is not consistent across genders. Monitoring for adverse effects, potential risks, and HT cessation is based on ongoing evaluations and determined on an individualized basis.[18]

- Common Screening and Risks Related to Testosterone Use between Men and TGD Men: Providers need to consider the commonalities of actual or potential risks and potential for underlying conditions before the initiation of testosterone therapy among cisgender and transgender men. Baseline screening includes age, and personal or family history of cardiovascular disease including CHF or other edematous-causing conditions, erythrocytosis, thrombosis, thrombophilia, stroke, smoking or alcohol use, and breast or reproductive organ cancer. Personal or family history of osteoporosis or metabolic disorder would also need to be considered on an individual basis before HT commencement.[30] If the man is considering fertility within the next 6 to 12 months, testosterone should be avoided. Following additional current screening recommendations based on individual and diverse backgrounds related to age, presence of reproductive organs, family and personal history, and lifestyle factors will assist clinical decision-making in the use and management of HT to avoid potential adverse effects.

- Testosterone Use Monitoring for Men and TGD Men: Monitoring serum testosterone, hematocrit, and hemoglobin levels should be done approximately every 3 months for the first year and every 6 to 12 months thereafter. Monitoring for adverse effects, potential risks, and HT cessation is based on ongoing evaluations and determined on an individualized basis.[5]

- Individualized Approach: With the wealth of knowledge and breakthroughs in genetic research, providers must consider how HT can affect the body under the influence of genetics, biological sex, and gender. There is consensus among medical societies, research, and current treatment guidelines for the emphasis of individualization in the decision to the initiation and management HT.[17] Initiation of HT including route, dosing, and duration should be made on an individualized basis after discussing the risks and benefits. HT benefits should be considered in the context of the overall health benefit, symptom control, and improvement of quality of life for the individual.[18] Overall, HT is considered safe, effective, and well tolerated by all people, regardless of sex or gender. Risks associated with HT in patients with TGD are comparable to those of patients with non-TGD.[5] Clinicians should be aware of gender-inclusive commonalities and offer a tailor approach to mitigate risks, prevent disease, and improve outcomes and quality of life, for all patients with HT needs.

- Further Research: The need for additional research on health care needs for TGD individuals is lacking regarding GAHT. Research on the long-term effects of estrogen and testosterone therapy in men, women, and TGD individuals is needed to increase gender-inclusive care and management of HT. Physiologic health benefits of GAHT such as improving mood, depression and well-being or prevention of CVD, osteoporosis, DM, and other conditions are not known, and research is needed in these areas.

## REFERENCES

1. Cagnacci A, Venier M. The Controversial History of Hormone Replacement Therapy. Medicina 2019;55(9):1–11.
2. Nieschlag E, Nieschlag S. Testosterone Deficiency: A Historical Perspective. Asian J Androl 2014;16(2):161–8.
3. Restar A, Jin H, Operario D. Gender – Inclusive and Gender – Specific Approaches in Trans Health Research. Transgender Health 2021;6(5):235–9.
4. World Health Organization. Gender and Health. 2021. Available at: https://www. who.int/news-room/questions-and-answers/item/gender-and-health. Accessed March 18, 2023.
5. Qian R, and Safer JD. Chapter 5: Hormone Treatment for the Adult Transgender Patient, In: Ferrando C., *Comprehensive care of the transgender patient*, 2020, Elsevier; Philidelphia, PA, 34–36.
6. Knudson G, Winter S, Baral S, et al. Chapter 1: An Introduction to Gender Diversity, In: Ferrando C.A., *Comprehensive care of the transgender patient*, 2020, Elsevier; Philidelphia, PA, 1–7.
7. Dwyer AA, Greenspan DL. Endocrine Nurses Society Position Statement on Transgender and Gender Diverse Care. Journal of the Endocrine Society 2021; 5(8):1–6. Available at: https://academic.oup.com/jes.
8. Thomas RL, Hirschhorn JN, and Majithia AR. Chapter 3: Genetics of Endocrinology, In: Melmed S., Williams *Textbook of endocrinology*, 14th edition, 2020, Elsevier; Philidelphia, PA, 42–61.
9. Chan Y-M, Hannema SE, Achermann JC, et al. Chapter 24: Disorders of Sex Deveopment, In: Melmed S., Williams *textbook of endocrinology*, 14th edition, 2020, Elsevier; Philidelphia, PA, 867–936.
10. Safer J, Tangpricha V. Care of Transgender Persons, *N Engl J Med*, 381 (25), 2019, 2451–2460.
11. Melmed S, Auchus RJ, Goldfine AB, et al. Chapter 1: Principles of Endocrinology, In: Melmed S., *Williams textbook of endocrinology*, 14th edition, 2020, Elsevier; Philidelphia, PA, 2–12.
12. Wolf-Gould C, Wolf-Gould C. Chapter 12: Primary and Preventative Care for Transgender Patients. In: Ferrando C, editor. Comprehensive care of the transgender patient. Philidelphia, PA: Elsevier; 2020. p. 114–30.
13. Bulun S. Chapter 17: Physiology and Pathology of the Female Reproductive Axis. In: Melmed S, editor. Williams textbook of endocrinology. 14th edition. Philidelphia, PA, Elsevier; 2020. p. 574–641.
14. Hewitt, Sylvia, et al. "Molecular Biology and Physiology of the Estrogen Action." Up To date. 2023. Available at: https://www-uptodate-com.www.remote.uwosh. edu/contents/molecular-biology-and-physiology-of-estrogen-action?search=e

strogen%20&source=search_result&selectedTitle=3~142&usage_type=default&display_rank=2#H2. Accessed March 19, 2023.

15. Matsumoto A, Anawalt BD. Chapter 19: Testicular Disorders. In: Melmed S, Williams, editors. *textbook of endocrinology*. 14th edition. Philadelphia, PA: Elsevier; 2020. p. 668–755.

16. Langer RD, Hodis HN, Lobo RA, et al. Hormone Replacement Therapy Where are We Now? Climacteric 2021;24(1):3–10.

17. Kim-Kyung J. Chapter 25: Estrogen: Impact on Cardiomyocytes and the Heart. In: Legato M, editor. Principles of gender-specific medicine. 3rd edition. Philidelphia, PA: Elsevier; 2017. p. 363–79.

18. Vigneswaran K, Hamoda H. Hormone Replacement Therapy – Current Recommendations. Best Pract Res Clin Obstet Gynaecol 2022;81:8–21.

19. Lobo RA. Chapter 14: Menopause and Aging. In: Jerome S, et al, editors. Yen & Jaffe's reproductive endocrinology. 8th edition. Philidelphia, PA, Elsevier; 2019. p. 322–56.

20. Hodis HN, Mack WJ. Menopausal Hormone Replacement Therapy and Reduction of All-Cause Mortality and Cardiovascular Disease: It's About Time and Timing. Cancer J 2022;28(3):208–23.

21. D'Alonzo M, Bounous VE, Villa M, et al. Current Evidence of the Oncological Benefit-Risk Profile of Hormone Replacement Therapy. Medicina 2019;55(573):1–7.

22. De Paula F, Black DM, Rosen CJ. Chapter 30: Osteoporosis: Basic and Clinical Aspects. In: Melmed S, editor. *Williams textbook of endocrinology*. 14th edition. Philidelphia, PA: Elsevier; 2020. p. 1256–97.

23. Martin, Kathryn, et al. "Treatment of Menopausal Symptoms with Hormone Therapy." Up To Date. 2023. Available at: https://www-uptodate-com.www.remote.uwosh.edu/contents/treatment-of-menopausal-symptoms-with-hormone-therapy?search=estrogen%20therapy&source=search_result&selectedTitle=2~146&usage_type=default&display_rank=1#H3178370787. Accessed March 19, 2023.

24. United States Preventative Services Task Force. Prediabetes and Type 2 Diabetes: Screening. 2021. Available at: https://www.uspreventiveservicestaskforce.org/uspstf/index.php/recommendation/screening-for-prediabetes-and-type-2-diabetes. Accessed March 19, 2023.

25. United States Preventative Services Task Force. January 11, 2016 Breast Cancer: Screening. Available at: https://www.uspreventiveservicestaskforce.org/uspstf/index.php/recommendation/breast-cancer-screening. Accessed March 19, 2023.

26. Barbonetti A, D'Andrea S, Francavilla S. Testosterone replacement therapy. Andrology 2020;8:1551–66.

27. Bhasin S, Brito JP, Cunningham GR, et al. Testosterone Therapy in Men with Hypogonadism: An Endocrine Society Clinical Practice Guideline. J Clin Endocrinol Metab 2018;103(5):1715–44.

28. Yabluchanskiy A, Tsitouras PD. Is Testosterone Replacement Therapy in Older Men Effective and Safe? Drugs Aging 2019;36(11):981–9.

29. Zschaebitz E, Bradley A, Olson S, et al. Primary Care Practice for Gender-Divers Patients Using Gender-Affirming Hormone Therapy. J Nurse Pract 2023;19:1–8.

30. Moravek MB. Gender-Affirming Hormone Therapy for Transgender Men. Clin Obstet Gynecol 2018;61(4):687–704.

31. Ray A, Fernstrum A, Mahran A, et al. Testosterone Therapy and Risk of Breast Cancer Development: a Systematic Review. Curr Opin Urol 2020;30(3):340–8.

32. Ibis S–S. Chapter 50: Gender-Specific Medicine in Pharmaceutical Drug Discovery and Development. In: Legato M, editor. Principles of gender-specific medicine. 3rd edition. Philadelphia, PA: Elsevier; 2017. p. 733–41.

# UNITED STATES POSTAL SERVICE®
## Statement of Ownership, Management, and Circulation
### (All Periodicals Publications Except Requester Publications)

| 1. Publication Title | 2. Publication Number | 3. Filing Date |
|---|---|---|
| NURSING CLINICS OF NORTH AMERICA | 598 – 960 | 9/18/2023 |

| 4. Issue Frequency | 5. Number of Issues Published Annually | 6. Annual Subscription Price |
|---|---|---|
| MAR, JUN, SEP, DEC | 4 | $163.00 |

7. Complete Mailing Address of Known Office of Publication (Not printer) (Street, city, county, state, and ZIP+4®)

ELSEVIER INC.
230 Park Avenue, Suite 800
New York, NY 10169

Contact Person
Malathi Samayan

Telephone (Include area code)
91-44-4299-4507

8. Complete Mailing Address of Headquarters or General Business Office of Publisher (Not printer)

ELSEVIER INC.
230 Park Avenue, Suite 800
New York, NY 10169

9. Full Names and Complete Mailing Addresses of Publisher, Editor, and Managing Editor (Do not leave blank)

Publisher (Name and complete mailing address)

DOLORES MELONI, ELSEVIER INC.
1600 JOHN F KENNEDY BLVD. SUITE 1600
PHILADELPHIA, PA 19103-2899

Editor (Name and complete mailing address)

KERRY HOLLAND, ELSEVIER INC.
1600 JOHN F KENNEDY BLVD. SUITE 1600
PHILADELPHIA, PA 19103-2899

Managing Editor (Name and complete mailing address)

PATRICK MANLEY, ELSEVIER INC.
1600 JOHN F KENNEDY BLVD. SUITE 1600
PHILADELPHIA, PA 19103-2899

10. Owner (Do not leave blank. If the publication is owned by a corporation, give the name and address of the corporation immediately followed by the names and addresses of all stockholders owning or holding 1 percent or more of the total amount of stock. If not owned by a corporation, give the names and addresses of the individual owners. If owned by a partnership or other unincorporated firm, give its name and address as well as those of each individual owner. If the publication is published by a nonprofit organization, give its name and address.)

| Full Name | Complete Mailing Address |
|---|---|
| WHOLLY OWNED SUBSIDIARY OF REED/ELSEVIER, US HOLDINGS | 1600 JOHN F KENNEDY BLVD. SUITE 1600 PHILADELPHIA, PA 19103-2899 |

11. Known Bondholders, Mortgagees, and Other Security Holders Owning or Holding 1 Percent or More of Total Amount of Bonds, Mortgages, or Other Securities. If none, check box. ▶ ☐ None

| Full Name | Complete Mailing Address |
|---|---|
| N/A | |

12. Tax Status (For completion by nonprofit organizations authorized to mail at nonprofit rates) (Check one)
The purpose, function, and nonprofit status of this organization and the exempt status for federal income tax purposes:
☒ Has Not Changed During Preceding 12 Months
☐ Has Changed During Preceding 12 Months (Publisher must submit explanation of change with this statement)

PS Form 3526, July 2014 [Page 1 of 4 (see instructions page 4)]  PSN: 7530-01-000-9931  PRIVACY NOTICE: See our privacy policy on www.usps.com.

| 13. Publication Title | 14. Issue Date for Circulation Data Below |
|---|---|
| NURSING CLINICS OF NORTH AMERICA | JUNE 2023 |

15. Extent and Nature of Circulation

| | | Average No. Copies Each Issue During Preceding 12 Months | No. Copies of Single Issue Published Nearest to Filing Date |
|---|---|---|---|
| a. Total Number of Copies (Net press run) | | 212 | 189 |
| b. Paid Circulation (By Mail and Outside the Mail) | (1) Mailed Outside-County Paid Subscriptions Stated on PS Form 3541 (Include paid distribution above nominal rate, advertiser's proof copies, and exchange copies) | 164 | 143 |
| | (2) Mailed In-County Paid Subscriptions Stated on PS Form 3541 (Include paid distribution above nominal rate, advertiser's proof copies, and exchange copies) | 0 | 0 |
| | (3) Paid Distribution Outside the Mails Including Sales Through Dealers and Carriers, Street Vendors, Counter Sales, and Other Paid Distribution Outside USPS® | 37 | 35 |
| | (4) Paid Distribution by Other Classes of Mail Through the USPS (e.g., First-Class Mail®) | 6 | 6 |
| c. Total Paid Distribution (Sum of 15b (1), (2), (3), and (4)) | | 207 | 184 |
| d. Free or Nominal Rate Distribution (By Mail and Outside the Mail) | (1) Free or Nominal Rate Outside-County Copies Included on PS Form 3541 | 4 | 4 |
| | (2) Free or Nominal Rate In-County Copies Included on PS Form 3541 | 0 | 0 |
| | (3) Free or Nominal Rate Copies Mailed at Other Classes Through the USPS (e.g. First-Class Mail) | 0 | 0 |
| | (4) Free or Nominal Rate Distribution Outside the Mail (Carriers or other means) | 1 | 1 |
| e. Total Free or Nominal Rate Distribution (Sum of 15d (1), (2), (3) and (4)) | | 5 | 5 |
| f. Total Distribution (Sum of 15c and 15e) | | 212 | 189 |
| g. Copies not Distributed (See Instructions to Publishers #4 (page 43)) | | 0 | 0 |
| h. Total (Sum of 15f and g) | | 212 | 189 |
| i. Percent Paid (15c divided by 15f times 100) | | 97.64% | 97.35% |

* If you are claiming electronic copies, go to line 16 on page 3. If you are not claiming electronic copies, skip to line 17 on page 3.

16. Electronic Copy Circulation

| | Average No. Copies Each Issue During Preceding 12 Months | No. Copies of Single Issue Published Nearest to Filing Date |
|---|---|---|
| a. Paid Electronic Copies ▶ | | |
| b. Total Paid Print Copies (Line 15c) + Paid Electronic Copies (Line 16a) ▶ | | |
| c. Total Print Distribution (Line 15f) + Paid Electronic Copies (Line 16a) ▶ | | |
| d. Percent Paid (Both Print & Electronic Copies) (16b divided by 16c × 100) ▶ | | |

☒ I certify that 99% of all my distributed copies (electronic and print) are paid above a nominal price.

17. Publication of Statement of Ownership
☒ If the publication is a general publication, publication of this statement is required. Will be printed
in the __DECEMBER 2023__ issue of this publication.  ☐ Publication not required.

18. Signature and Title of Editor, Publisher, Business Manager, or Owner

*Malathi Samayan*   Date 9/18/2023

Malathi Samayan - Distribution Controller

I certify that all information furnished on this form is true and complete. I understand that anyone who furnishes false or misleading information on this form or who omits material or information requested on the form may be subject to criminal sanctions (including fines and imprisonment) and/or civil sanctions (including civil penalties).

PS Form 3526, July 2014 (Page 3 of 4)  PRIVACY NOTICE: See our privacy policy on www.usps.com

# *Moving?*

## Make sure your subscription moves with you!

To notify us of your new address, find your **Clinics Account Number** (located on your mailing label above your name), and contact customer service at:

Email: **journalscustomerservice-usa@elsevier.com**

**800-654-2452** (subscribers in the U.S. & Canada)
**314-447-8871** (subscribers outside of the U.S. & Canada)

**Fax number: 314-447-8029**

**Elsevier Health Sciences Division**
**Subscription Customer Service**
**3251 Riverport Lane**
**Maryland Heights, MO 63043**

*To ensure uninterrupted delivery of your subscription, please notify us at least 4 weeks in advance of move.